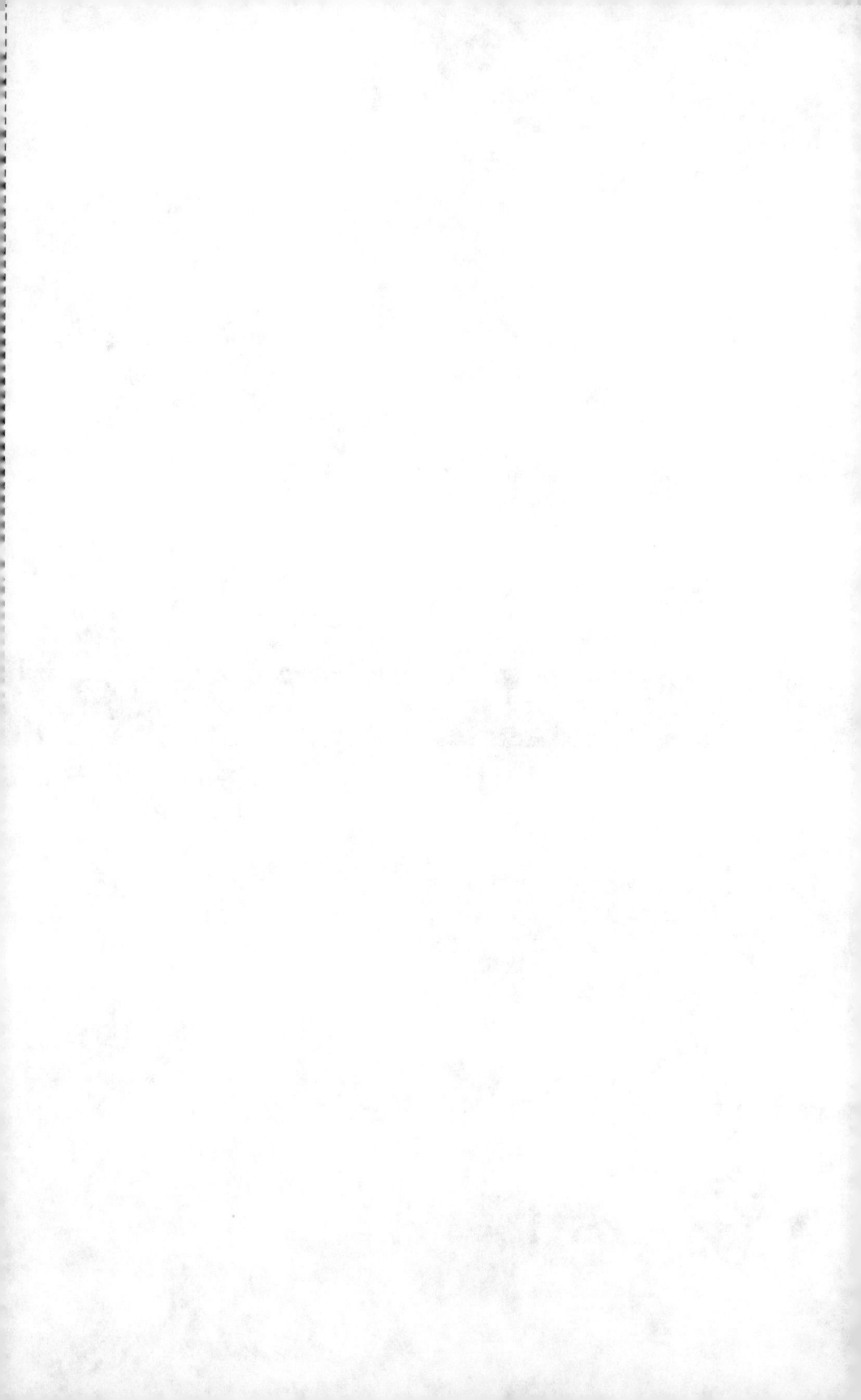

UNDERSTANDING
PTSD

UNDERSTANDING
PTSD

Austin Mardon, PhD

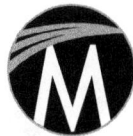

MERCURY LEARNING AND INFORMATION
Boston, Massachusetts

Publisher: David Pallai
MERCURY LEARNING AND INFORMATION
121 High Street, 3rd Floor
Boston, MA 02110
info@merclearning.com
www.merclearning.com
800-232-0223

A. Mardon. *Understanding PTSD.*
ISBN: 978-1-50152-287-1

The publisher recognizes and respects all marks used by companies, manufacturers, and developers as a means to distinguish their products. All brand names and product names mentioned in this book are trademarks or service marks of their respective companies. Any omission or misuse (of any kind) of service marks or trademarks, etc. is not an attempt to infringe on the property of others.

Library of Congress Control Number: 2024940391

242526321   This book is printed on acid-free paper in the United States of America.

Our titles are available for adoption, license, or bulk purchase by institutions, corporations, etc. For additional information, please contact the Customer Service Dept. at 800-232-0223 (toll free).

To

My beloved spouse

CONTENTS

INTRODUCTION: *A COLLEGE STUDENT'S STORY*

S amantha was an above average student; ambitious and driven to succeed in every aspect of her life. She discovered that in order to succeed she had to have a loving and secure relationship with those closest to her. At the time, Samantha's closest connections were with her parents, younger sister, and brother, as well as her long-term boyfriend. Throughout high school she would often volunteer her time at local nonprofit organizations as well as help out at homeless shelters around her immediate location. After graduation, Samantha prepared to depart for university; she was full of excitement and passion for what lay ahead of her. Despite her sadness at leaving those she loved behind; she told her loved ones that she would stay connected by writing letters and calling as often as possible to try and make the time pass between them smoother and quicker.

When Samantha started school, she immediately expressed extraordinary interest in her psychology course. Her textbooks were full of theories and explanations on learning, emotions, and memory that she seemed to never want to put down. Samantha would spend hours in the library and in her dorm reading and analyzing her books, absorbing all the information she could in a small amount of time.

It was a five-block walk from Samantha's dorm to the library. One night she left the library just before closing time around 1 o'clock in the morning. On this night in particular, she was in a rush to get home so she decided that she could save some time if she would cut through the back alley behind a few buildings before returning onto the path to her dorm.

As she took this shortcut through the back alley, a dark shape came alive from the shadows and a man's bulky and strong figure seemed to block all the space in front of her. Samantha tried to run, but there was no escaping the menacing figure before her. He was too strong, and she couldn't injure him in any way; he simply overpowered her, leaving her feeling helpless with no hope, alone, and surrounded by darkness. The assailant took a strong hold of her, covered her mouth, and whispered in her ear, "Don't make a sound, or this will end worse than it started." The man released his hold on her face and smacked her across her mouth, proceeding to rape her and then he let her drop to the cold hard cement when he was done. Samantha lay crumpled on the ground with no understanding of time or space, only that all she felt was fear and a sense of being lost. All she could think was that his breath smelled like caramel.

Samantha felt like she had become damaged goods after that night; her philosophy of human nature had forever changed, and she could no longer believe the theories that she once read from her beloved textbooks. Not only was her body scratched and altered, but so was her identity. After that night, Samantha's sense of trust was taken from her, that night where she felt uncertain and lost in a world she now viewed as dangerous and full of terror.

Samantha's grades suffered; she could not find the motivation to study the things that she once believed in with no reservations. She no longer had a relationship with her family members, and she lost her boyfriend in the process. After that night, Samantha could not communicate about her daily activities and experiences. She could not share her story of what happened that night to those she cared about, and she could no longer relate to those around her. Samantha became haunted and terrorized by every shadow. In every dark corner and alley, she saw the same menacing figure from that night. She was so frightened that she no longer left her room at night, regardless of whether others would be accompanying her. She became so obsessed with her attacker that she soon found excuses to not leave her room in the daylight. She began to hide from the world around her, and she only felt safe in her own room. Even then, at night the attacker would return to her in her dreams, where she believed he had come to finish the job he started in that dark alley. To this day the smell of caramel makes her curl into the fetal position and wait for the memory to end.

Samantha is suffering from posttraumatic stress disorder (PTSD).

As you can see from Samantha's story, posttraumatic stress disorder is not as cut and dry as the media and other modern resources have made it out to be. In most cases, society has been led to believe PTSD is only experienced by war veterans or those exposed to war zone areas. Unfortunately, this is not the truth. Posttraumatic stress disorder, better known as PTSD, can be experienced by anyone that has been exposed to a traumatic event, regardless of where it took place. Trauma has been defined in regard to this condition as anything that causes an individual to feel fear, stress, anxiety, or loss of control.

It is important to understand that this book has not been written for an academic audience, rather that it has been specifically designed for the general population. This means that a lot of the technical jargon has been removed when explaining what PTSD is and how it affects individuals. It was important for the author to try and explain PTSD in a way that could be understood by everyone. This is essential, because in many cases when people try to explain mental disorders and conditions, people end up being more confused than before they read the explanation. This does more harm than good because people ignore the explanations they do not understand, and they instead simply pick out the information that they can understand. In an attempt to clarify PTSD, the authors of this book took a simplistic approach to explaining PTSD. Each of the chapters has been broken down into subsections, where these smaller sections of the chapters take the time to explain in nontechnical words what each of the elements are.

Before we dive into the book, it is important to try and get a feel for what PTSD is. As you know, this condition and its symptoms are brought on by a traumatic event. In most cases where PTSD has been developed within an individual, they surround themselves in the belief that it is either their fault or that it was the fault of someone else. In the case of Samantha, it is extremely likely that she will blame herself for being in the situation. It is also possible that those around her will also blame her and say that nothing would have happened had she not put herself in harm's way in the first place. This is an extremely common scenario that tends to play out when people acknowledge that they are now suffering from PTSD.

Another quite common situation is that when people feel shame or guilt, they will not seek help from anyone, be it a professional or someone they are close to. In cases where people do not try and get help, the symptoms of PTSD begin to take over the individual's life. This causes them to pull away from those that are trying to help them through whatever it is that they are feeling. The individual then puts up a wall between themself and those around them.

The barrier acts as their protection against the feelings associated with PTSD. This is the wall that many individuals hide behind to avoid talking about their trauma and "forgetting" the trauma ever occurred. Unfortunately, by ignoring the trauma and the associated symptoms, their condition worsens.

The goal for this book is to educate those who don't know much about PTSD. By educating individuals on PTSD, it is not only about learning about a disorder, but it is about teaching people how to adjust to life with PTSD. This book will help those not only directly affected by PTSD but those being affected indirectly.

One major cause for individuals avoiding help is shame. Victims feel shame because they now have to live with this condition, and the shame that the media has led them to believe that they are flawed and that it is why they are now living with a condition. In many cases the media has stated that PTSD is caused by an individual either being crazy or even weak-minded. Fortunately, as society becomes more informed of PTSD and by understanding their circumstances, these individuals will hopefully be more inclined to seek help from those around them as well as from professional resources if needed. Reading a book like this is the first step in a victim's attempt to help their situation.

Another goal of this book is to educate those around a victim of PTSD. It is vital that the victim personally understands what they are going through. But it is of equal importance for bystanders to understand the truth behind the disorder. When those around the victim acknowledge what is going on, they can then take specific steps to help them work through their issues. It also gives the victim a confidant without having to go public with their PTSD. It allows them to take the first step in admitting that there is something wrong.

Before you read more of this book, it's important to know that PTSD is an overwhelmingly difficult disorder to deal with. Nonetheless, it is not an impossible task to learn to deal with, and even defeat, symptoms associated with PTSD. If you are someone that has PTSD and you are reading this book, remember that things will get better, but not without working to make things better. For those reading this book who are witnesses to someone dealing with PTSD, you have to support the sufferer of PTSD in whatever they do, as long as it is not harming them. It is vital to be there for them, let them know that everything is going to be alright, and that you will be there for them no matter what.

CHAPTER 1

THE HISTORY OF PSYCHOTRAUMATOLOGY

Posttraumatic stress disorder (PTSD) is said to be a relatively new psychological disorder, but in actuality, PTSD has simply become a new title for a very old condition. Symptoms of PTSD can be identified going back as far as three thousand years ago, to the time of an Egyptian named Hori who once wrote about the fear and anxiety with descriptions of shaking and raised hair. It was believed that Hori wrote about these symptoms in regard to his experiences in past battles ("What Is PTSD?," 2024). Although this description does not specifically fit the criteria for PTSD, it does have similar symptoms of what would be a part of a current medical explanation of PTSD.

Here are just a few of the titles or "nicknames" that have been given for PTSD over the years. Some of the more common names that most veterans know this condition is either Soldier's Heart or Da Costa's Syndrome. This was discovered and named by an internal medicine doctor by the name of Jacob Mendez, who studied Civil War veterans in the United States and identified that many of these soldiers were suffering from chest-thumping, anxiety, and shortness of breath.

PTSD IN HISTORICAL TEXTS

Long before PTSD was an official psychological diagnosis, it was still often able to be recognized. Soldiers or civilians alike, after witnessing the trauma of others or enduring their own, displayed a similar array of symptoms captured in centuries of poetry, art, official records, myths, and personal journals. People would display symptoms of injury, such as blindness, despite not being physically harmed, and would be wracked with nightmares or illusions of a previous traumatic experience.

One of the earliest known records of PTSD-like symptoms dates back to 1300–609 BC, when ancient Mesopotamians faced many wars. The citizens' trauma manifested as difficulty sleeping, as well as invasive memories of the destruction they had witnessed. Observations by Herodotus note the psychological struggles of Epizelus after his time at war in 490 BC. Appian of Alexandria also described a veteran who burned down his own home with himself in it as a defense against the oncoming threat of battle against his village. Furthermore, *Life of Marius* by Plutarch tells of Caius Marius and his struggles with sleep, substance abuse, and flashbacks, which are comparable to currently known symptoms of PTSD (Shipp, 2022). While these instances cannot be confirmed to be the PTSD we know today, they do point to similar symptoms and experiences, which works to reveal how the illness, or forms of it, have been around for at least as long as humans could leave records for people to find.

Documentation of the Hundred Years' War in England and France revealed how soldiers struggled with anxieties and nightmares related to their experiences in battle ("History of PTSD," n.d.). Samuel Pepys (1633–1703) was an English naval administrator and member of Parliament whose valuable diary captured both key moments of upper-class life, and the Fire of London in 1666 (Bryant, 2024). He wrote about the fire in the time after it ended, where he included information about the struggles of survivors, as well as his own struggles, which included sleep riddled with recurring nightmares of the great fire which destroyed much of London (Bryant, 2024). Though no one took the time to diagnose and treat Pepys for PTSD, the repetitive nature of his nightmares are consistent with PTSD symptoms still experienced today. As such, his valuable account of life in seventeenth-century London works to further emphasize that PTSD is far older than its label would indicate.

Literature and art also capture a great historical interest in understanding the symptoms of PTSD. Soldiers having recurring nightmares of battles appear in tales such as Homer's *Iliad* and the works of Shakespeare (Chicco and Tebala 2020; "History of PTSD," n.d.). The *Gisli Súrsson Saga*, an Icelandic story estimated to have been written during the thirteenth century, recounts how the hero Gisli suffers from vivid nightmares of battle, so much so that he cannot safely rest alone and fears sleeping (Larson, 2021). In the epic poem *The Epic of Gilgamesh*, Gilgamesh himself endures flashbacks of the death of his close companion. He is wrought with questions about his own death and his guilt (de Villiers, 2020). The Bible clarifies that in some cases, this pattern of soldiers losing sleep or being permanently affected by battlefield trauma was recognized not just by diarists and poets but by military leaders. They also recognized the way that one soldier's psychological symptoms may affect others. The Book of Deuteronomy in the Old Testament provides the advice of letting traumatized men go home, rather than risk the hearts of his comrades, as well as his own (Janzen, 2019. These examples combine to show the ubiquity of PTSD symptoms, revealing that they are so common they enter into stories and histories throughout time.

EVOLVING TERMS DURING BATTLE

PTSD symptoms, especially on the battlefield, underwent centuries of medical misdiagnosis and general confusion from physicians. Soldiers with the disorder were often treated alongside, and confused with, cases of traumatic brain injury (TBI), as both had a lack of apparent physical injury and had similar symptoms. In time, psychotraumatology would split as a subspecialty from traumatology, but it would first endure a long series of ever-changing names, definitions, and euphemisms as militaries addressed this extremely common and debilitating disorder in their troops (Jongedijk et al., 2023).

Swiss doctor Johannes Hofer in his 1688 medical dissertation championed the next most notable name, *nostalgia*. This name survived until the end of the Seven Years War. Hofer classified the disorder as consisting of depression, angst, and both physical and mental exhaustion. Due to the increased interest in the soldier's medical conditions, other medical sources began to argue that these symptoms of nostalgia were not in relation to an actual battlefield experience, but that it was in association with the soldier's longing to return home, due to being apart from their loved ones for extended campaigns. French and German doctors took these soldiers classified with nostalgia and instead identified them as having *homesickness*. This then led to Spain creating their own way of identifying these individuals, where these same symptoms of PTSD became known as *estar roto*, which means "to be broken." This new construct for PTSD lasted for another sixteen years throughout the length of the Napoleonic era (1799–1816).

As you can see there have been numerous names for PTSD. Interestingly, throughout the years, researchers only identified PTSD as being related to war soldiers. The written history of PTSD centered on the belief that only soldiers experienced a great enough trauma to suffer from PTSD. This has led contemporary society to continue to believe in the myth that only war veterans are affected by PTSD.

In the late 1700s, civilian PTSD appeared in great numbers for the first time, as a consequence of the Industrial Revolution. Due to increased mechanizations, disasters were at a scale and of a type rarely seen by civilians. Charles Dickens wrote about witnessing the death of people during a railway accident, which led to his phobia of traveling by train. In the late 1800s, the famous author Charles Dickens was involved in a railway accident in Staplehurst in Kent England. Dickens later wrote about his experiences and symptoms, claiming that he believed they were associated with the railway accident. He wrote in a letter explaining the horrifying scene he experienced, as well as stating that he did not feel himself, and believed this to be a result of the railway accident (Perdue, 2022). It was these instances that led to more social belief that PTSD could be caused by more than just killing or witnessing people being killed.

The railway accidents introduced the diagnoses "railway spine," as some believed survivors suffered microscopic damage to the spine and brain. English surgeon John Eric Erichsen blamed this in particular on spinal concussions with the assertion that even in the absence of a fracture, physical damage from the accident caused inflammation in the spinal cord and subsequent psychological symptoms (Gasquoine, 2020). Due to the fact that PTSD was not in existence for anyone other than war soldiers, no one understood what Dickens was going through at the time. As we read about this today, we know that what he must have been feeling is a direct description of modern-day PTSD. Unfortunately, in the 1800s, people chose not to believe this theory of trauma that caused physical and mental ailments within individuals. After multiple railway accidents, people started to sue the companies stating that there was something unknown that started to happen to them after the accidents. Lawyers of the railways said the litigants were trying to get something from nothing, due to so many people discounting the effects of trauma. They stated that this supposed trauma only affected individuals with ulterior motives such as money, food, and shelter. Following the aftermath of this, people started considering the idea that PTSD symptoms could come from situations outside of the military world. Unfortunately, PTSD was left out of any sort of medical description not involving soldiers.

Meanwhile, battlefields still saw soldiers with trouble sleeping, anxiety, and a wish to return home. Austrian physician Josef Leopold called this *"nostalgia,"* a term that would linger into the Civil War. The aforementioned French physician who treated the man with nightmares of drowning also treated patients during the French Revolution. He called this collection of familiar symptoms "cardiorespiratory neurosis" or "idiotism" ("History of PTSD," n.d.; Zhou et al., 2021). During the French Revolution and the Napoleonic wars, "vent du boulet" (the wind of the ball) syndrome often explained why soldiers became inconsolable after being nearly hit by cannonballs (Jongedijk et al., 2023). Today, "sentir le vent du boulet" (literally "feeling the wind of the cannonball") is a French idiom expressing relief at narrowly escaping danger ("Sentir le Vent du Boulet," n.d.). Johann Wolfgang Goethe, German poet and survivor of the 1792 battle of Valmy, described soldiers who seemed to be catatonic after battle attacks. He refers to the experience of the battlefield as a hot and scary place, with a change in hue and feeling which gave the feeling that it was consumed in fire (Dollar, 2022). The struggles of Napoleonic soldiers prove the struggle to survive severe trauma and highlights yet another turn in society's understanding of PTSD.

The Civil War brought the term *"irritable heart"* to the forefront of social understanding. Soldiers reported rapid or irregular heartbeats, headaches, trouble sleeping, physical imbalance, anxiety, and a lack of concentration. There is no definitive proof whether irritable heart was truly a form of PTSD, or instead a related *"conversion disorder,"* wherein psychological distress manifests as physical symptoms (Dollar,

2022; Mayo Clinic Staff, 2022). Regardless of possible alternatives, it is worth noting the similarities between the experiences of Civil War soldiers and soldiers today who suffer with PTSD.

The decades after the Civil War caused further confusion in understanding PTSD. This occurred as physicians struggled to match symptoms with their proposed diagnoses and parse its complexity from other syndromes such as TBI. Civil War army surgeon Jacob Mendez da Costa used the term *"soldier's heart"* to describe a link between severe trauma and an increased risk of cardiovascular disease. Occasionally, sufferers of a soldier's heart would also experience paralysis or loss of sensation following the traumatic event (Bremner et al., 2020). French neurologist Jean-Martin Charcot proposed a concept of traumatic hysteria, adding that soldiers may be more likely to develop PTSD-like symptoms after a traumatic event depending on genetic factors. Charcot also noted the significance between past psychological traumas, disturbing dreams, and hysterical episodes (Bogousslavsky, 2020). In 1885, surgeon Henry Page reported that these symptoms were only psychological with no relation to spinal injury, and yet still caused the body's nervous system to malfunction. His chosen terms were *nervous shock* and *functional disorder*. German physician Hermann Oppenheim was the first to use the term *traumatic neurosis*. Traumatic neurosis would later be connected to a set of recognizable and specific PTSD symptoms, such as the requirement of trauma, dissociation caused by the trauma, and the role of pathogens within lost memories (Jongedijk et al., 2023; "History of PTSD and Trauma Diagnoses," n.d.). The idea that a person may be genetically predisposed to traumatic neurosis was later discarded. Unfortunately, Jean-Martin Charcot's criticisms that Oppenheim was simply redefining hysteria and hysteria-related syndromes would not allow the term to truly permeate French psychiatry until Charcot's death, showing the long battle to define the psychological effects of traumatic stressors. In 1889, American neurologist George Miller Beard classified under "neurasthenia" or "nervous exhaustion," symptoms such as inability to sleep, lethargy, headaches, and depressive feelings. Anemia was also blamed during the turn of the century, at fault for syndromes called "disorderly action of the heart" and "irritability of the heart." Morgan Fincuane brought railway spine to the battlefield after the Boer War, noting that much like railway accident survivors, soldiers with these syndromes had continuous, psychologically related nerve and muscle problems even after their wounds healed ("History of PTSD and Trauma Diagnoses," n.d.). Despite the numerous names and considerations, it is clear that doctors and scientists have been exploring similar symptoms noted for soldiers and war survivors throughout history.

PTSD IN THE WORLD WARS

Regardless of the terms being used to diagnose the soldiers, most militaries across various wars would take affected soldiers away from the battlefield to treat them in an environment of relative peace and normalcy. During the Civil War, a psychiatric hospital was created to handle the increasing quantity of cases, but in time, they moved patients from the apparent death sentence of battlefield care to their homes. In 1904–1905 however, Charles S. Myers helped develop the idea of "forward psychiatric treatment," which kept soldiers close to the front lines during treatment: this concept would evolve throughout World War I and II, until becoming standard practice in the modern day (Johnson, 2021). Forward treatment, or "forward psychiatry," was specifically for stress-related issues. Surprisingly, soldiers who were treated within reach of both their comrades and the sounds of battle more reliably recovered from their symptoms. It appeared that remaining within the military hierarchy setting would stave off the chronic disability that evacuated patients developed. Forward treatment's five principles were: immediacy (treating soldiers immediately, which may prevent chronic symptoms), proximity (treatment near the front line rather than an environment of quiet and peace), expectancy (communicating to the patient that recovery was imminent), simplicity (simple treatment such as rest), and centrality (all medical personnel following the same rules and ideals) (Zhou et al., 2021). For these soldiers, Forward treatment became an important feature of traumatic stress treatment which carried forward to future wars.

Nonetheless, the conflict of interest between military leaders and their soldiers, whose diagnoses were, throughout the wars, rife with controversy and accusations of cowardice, must be considered when describing the success of forward treatment. Among the contentious and contradictory discussions of PTSD in both soldiers and citizens, there were those who did not believe that symptoms of PTSD were actually medical. During the late 1800s in Prussia, new compensation laws for railway accidents appeared to infect many with "compensation neurosis," who then applied for disability status. A study by a German psychiatrist, Bonhoeffer, in 1926 claimed nearly all soldiers with traumatic neurosis were simply seeking health insurance payouts, and as a result, Germany pulled their compensation for these veterans ("History of PTSD and Trauma Diagnoses," n.d.). PTSD appeared to only be a manifestation of a "deficiency of character," which resulted in the execution of many soldiers for desertion or other such supposed crimes ("Shot at Dawn," 2021). This prompted a tangle of treatments, different diagnoses, and attempts by militaries and physicians to keep enough soldiers healthy while not losing too many of their numbers to these inscrutable disorders.

Soldiers were then said to suffer from *shell shock*, an umbrella term that today appears to cover a combination of PTSD and TBI. The term arose most frequently when soldiers were near, but untouched by, explosions. Of British military, there were over 250,000 soldiers who were diagnosed with shell shock (The National Archives, n.d.). Shell shock, and its eventual encapsulation of many psychological disorders, recognized serious and potentially treatable problems. Soldiers eventually became less nervous about revealing their symptoms only to be accused of a weakness of character. As cases skyrocketed, the military struggled to maintain both treatment and their fighting numbers. Unfortunately, the diagnosis "hysteria" returned as well as the idea that this was not caused by combat but instead by a preexisting personality disorder. Governments did not have to pay disability in such cases. British psychiatrists at times referred to these cases as simply stress-related and officially "not yet diagnosed, nervous," and returned the soldiers to the field (Park et al., 2022). This would, of course, create a lot of ambiguity around the progressing understanding of PTSD.

World War II saw a great change in military and medical opinions of PTSD. Symptoms in survivors were extensively studied and psychiatrists introduced psychological assessments and screening tests in military applicants. Unfortunately, preexisting psychological conditions could not reliably predict the development of PTSD. Psychiatric casualties were better recognized, however, as was the importance of the stress of battle on a soldier's risk of developing PTSD. Studies eventually provided data revealing that 20%–50% of discharges in the World War II military were considered to be psychiatric in nature ("History of PTSD and Trauma Diagnoses," n.d.). A 1946 report concluded that psychiatric casualties were as common as gunshot casualties, and that the time in which a soldier achieved the highest level of efficacy was within his first ninety days at battle. It was also found that 98% of soldiers developed psychiatric symptoms of some kind after sixty days of battle (Gnam, 2023). The epidemic was clearly widespread and for many decades very difficult to track and understand, but this data became key in defining new regulations during later wars. Forward treatment returned to the forefront, with 50%-70% of those with psychiatric syndromes returning to duty (Gnam, 2023).

Traumatic neurosis was the popular term for civilian PTSD symptoms. In 1941, it was concluded that the aforementioned assortment of terms in the military were all the same syndrome under different monikers, promoting a consistency that was much needed within the field ("History of PTSD and Trauma Diagnoses," n.d.). After the war, a Russian psychiatry textbook collected many of the terms under one umbrella: *affective shock reactions*. These were related to traumatic events such as war, natural disasters, or the ever-popular railway accidents, and manifest as psychological symptoms lasting either a few days or a few months (Zhou et al., 2021).

World War II also allowed the study of PTSD in civilians rather than only soldiers. Many civilians had lived under occupation of enemy forces, endured torture, or been imprisoned in concentration camps. Some experienced a decline in health over a long period of time. Among the longitudinal data, there were yet more terms such as *concentration camp syndrome*, which was described as a process of rapid aging where patients showed emotional issues, extreme lethargy, and mental and physical decline ("History of PTSD and Trauma Diagnoses," n.d.). By the end of the Vietnam War, data collected revealed that out of the 2.7 million people the United States sent to war, 700,000 of them were in need of psychiatric care (Godwin, 2021). After decades of new names, in 1980, the term *posttraumatic stress disorder* officially entered the third edition of the *Diagnostic and Statistical Manual of Mental Disorders* (Godwin, 2021). When the book was first published, there was a lot of controversy surrounding its factuality in the medical world. As more people started to understand the symptoms and elements of the onset of PTSD, it was believed that PTSD was actually filling in a gap that had existed in the psychiatric theory. As more extensive research was compiled on PTSD, it was found that in order for the symptoms of PTSD to come into effect, trauma has to occur. As stated earlier, this trauma was once said to be an inherent internal weakness of the individual, but it is now known that trauma occurs because of an external event. This definition was preceded by various adjustments, additions, and addendums, but it had found its name and with it, the scientific field of psychotraumatology (Ozturk et al., 2021). The definition includes diagnostic criteria that encapsulates both civilian and military trauma. Research continues to develop in order to more accurately capture the disorder and define effective treatments, which will be expanded upon in the following chapters.

In conclusion, PTSD is one of the most unique psychiatric disorders to diagnose because most of the emphasis is placed upon identifying what sort of traumatic stressor has occurred. This is essential because a professional PTSD diagnosis cannot be made without the individual meeting the specific stressor criteria. This means that the trauma they experience has to be identifiable as a traumatic event. For example, some forms of trauma have been identified as rape, physical violence, natural disaster, mental harassment, and war zone trauma. It is important to note that a lot of controversy surrounds PTSD because individuals find it hard to comprehend how everyone does not become a victim of PTSD. They wonder how it is that multiple people can experience the exact same traumatic event yet not all of the individuals involved suffer from PTSD. Though there is no distinct medical explanation as to why this happens, it is believed that PTSD is related to historical events in the individual's past. This simply means that the experiences and events that an individual has gone through in the past prior to the actual traumatic event has an effect on how people will react to the current trauma. In some cases, this means that if an individual has never experienced a traumatic event in their life, they will be less inclined to suffer from severe symptoms associated with PTSD. Whereas if an individual has been exposed to other traumas in their past, by experiencing another trauma it can cause a domino effect of the new trauma, releasing the strong emotions and symptoms that were associated with the first trauma. This unfortunately causes the PTSD victim to almost suffer from two or more traumas at the same time, which intensifies the severe symptoms of PTSD.

REFERENCES

Bougousslavsky, J. "The Mysteries of Hysteria: A Historical Perspective." *International Review of Psychiatry* 32, no. 5–6: 437–50, May 19, 2020. https://doi.org/10.1080/09540261.2020.1772731.

Brenmer, J. D., M. T. Wittbrodt, A. J. Shah, B. D. Pearce, N. Z. Gurel, O. T. Inan, P. Raggi, T. T. Lewis, A. A. Quyyumi, and V. Vaccarino. "Confederates in the Attic: Posttraumatic Stress Disorder, Cardiovascular Disease, and the Return of Soldier's Heart." *Journal of Nervous & Mental Disease* 208, no. 3: 171–80, March 2020. https://doi.org/10.1097/nmd.0000000000001100.

Bryant, A. "Samuel Pepys." *Encyclopedia Britannica*, February 2, 2024. https://www.britannica.com/biography/Samuel-Pepys

Chicco, M., and G. D. Tebala. "War Trauma in Homer's Iliad: A Trauma Registry Perspective." *European Journal of Trauma and Emergency Surgery* 47, no. 3: 773–78, April 18, 2020. https://doi.org/10.1007/s00068-020-01365-6

de Villiers, G. "Suffering in the Epic of Gilgamesh." *Old Testament Essays* 33, no. 3: 690–705, 2020. https://doi.org/10.17159/2312-3621/2020/v33n3a19

Dollar, E. A. *Hearts Torn Asunder: Trauma in the Civil War's Final Campaign in North Carolina*. Savas Beatie, 2022.

Gasquoine, P. G. "Railway Spine: The Advent of Compensation for Concussive Symptoms." *Journal of the History of Neurosciences* 29, no. 2: 234–45, January 27, 2020. https://doi:10.1080/0964704X.2019.1711350

Gnam, C. "Combat Fatigue: How Stress in Battle Was Felt (and Treated) in WWII." Warfare History Network, October 17, 2023. https://warfarehistorynetwork.com/combat-fatigue-how-stress-in-battle-was-felt-and-treated-in-wwii/

Godwin, M. "How Veterans Created PTSD." *JSTOR Daily*, November 9, 2021. https://daily.jstor.org/how-veterans-created-ptsd/

"History of PTSD." Black Bear Lodge, n.d. https://blackbearrehab.com/mental-health/ptsd/history-of-ptsd/

"History of PTSD and Trauma Diagnoses." TraumaDissociation.com, n.d. http://traumadissociation.com/ptsd/history-of-post-traumatic-stress-disorder.html

Janzen, D. "Claimed and Unclaimed Experience: Problematic Readings of Trauma in the Hebrew Bible." *Biblical Interpretation* 27, no. 2: 163–85, May 8, 2019. https://doi.org/10.1163/15685152-00272p01.

Johnson, S. "How Psychiatric Ideas About Trauma Evolved After World War I." Big Think, September 21, 2021. https://bigthink.com/mind-brain/trauma-evolution-psychiatry/.

Jongedijk, R. A., P. A., Boelen, J. W. Knipscheer, and R. J. Kleber. "Unity or Anarchy? A Historical Search for the Psychological Consequences of Psychotrauma." *Review of General Psychology* 27, no. 3: 303–19, February 23, 2023. https://doi.org/10.1177/10892680231153096

Larson, M. "Evolutionary Insights into a Maladapted Viking in Gísla Saga." Scholarly Publishing Collective, April 1, 2021. https://scholarlypublishingcollective.org/jegp/article-lookup/doi/10.5406/jenglgermphil.120.2.0141

Mayo Clinic Staff. "Functional Neurologic Disorder/Conversion Disorder." Mayo Clinic, January 11, 2022. https://www.mayoclinic.org/diseases-conditions/conversion-disorder/symptoms-causes/syc-20355197

The National Archives. "War Office Report on 'Shell shock.'" n.d. https://www.nationalarchives.gov.uk/education/resources/medicine-on-the-western-front-part-two/war-office-report-on-shell-shock/

Ozturk, E., B. Erdogan, and G. Derin. "Psychotraumatology and Dissociation: A Theoretical and Clinical Approach." *Medicine Science | International Medical Journal* 10, no. 1: 246–54, February 2021. https://doi.org/10.5455/medscience.2021.02.041

Park, J., L. Neilson, and A. K. Demetriades. "Hysteria, Head Injuries, and Heredity: 'Shell-Shocked' Soldiers of the Royal Edinburgh Asylum, Edinburgh (1914–24)." *Notes and Records: The Royal Society Journal of the History of Science* 77, no. 3: 443–70, March 2, 2022. https://doi.org/10.1098/rsnr.2021.0057

Perdue, D. A. "Charles Dickens, Henry Benge, and the Great Staplehurst Railway Crash." The Charles Dickens Page, April 8, 2022. https://www.charlesdickenspage.com/staplehurst-railway-crash-1865.html "Sentir Le Vent Du Boulet." Sentir le Vent du Boulet : Signification et Origine de l'Expression, n.d. https://www.linternaute.fr/expression/langue-francaise/19078/sentir-le-vent-du-boulet/.

Shipp, W. "How Did Ancient Warriors Deal with Post Traumatic Stress Disorder?" Australian Army Research Center, February 17, 2022. https://researchcentre.army.gov.au/library/land-power-forum/how-did-ancient-warriors-deal-post-traumatic-stress-disorder

"Shot at Dawn." Key Military, July 20, 2021. https://www.keymilitary.com/article/shot-dawn

"What Is PTSD?" Wounded Spirits Ministries, 2024. https://woundedspirits.com/what-is-ptsd/

Zhou, Y., Z. Shang, F. Zhang, L. Wu, L. Sun, Y. Jia, H. Yu, and W. Liu. "PTSD: Past, Present and Future Implications for China." *Chinese Journal of Traumatology* 24, no. 4: 187–208, July 2021. https://doi.org/10.1016/j.cjtee.2021.04.011

CHAPTER 2

PTSD Myths

O ver the years, the belief that PTSD is only experienced by combat soldiers who have been exposed to violence in war zones has grown. This has been the major belief for hundreds of years because symptoms of PTSD would most obviously be seen in those who have witnessed violence for a period of time. As more research is being done on PTSD, it has been recognized that the disorder has the ability to affect anyone with the experience of a traumatic event (Howard, 2024). For example, a traumatic event can be a car accident, various types of abuse or assault, a highly stressful event, or natural disaster. One of the major reasons why there have been misrepresentations of PTSD is because of the lack of information about why PTSD only affects select people among multiple individuals with the same experience. This is because there are a variety of ways in which people react to these specific traumatic events. It also has to do with past experiences the individual has had in life (Karstoft and Armour, 2022). This chapter goes through a list of some of the most famous misconceptions and misrepresentations of PTSD and explains why people have come to believe the misinformation, and why they should not believe it. It disputes the claims in an attempt to get individuals to try and understand more about this disorder. By understanding what PTSD is and how people interpret it, the reader as a knowledgeable individual will be able to try and provide assistance and support for victims suffering from this PTSD.

ONLY THE WEAK GET PTSD

Susceptibility has absolutely nothing to do with an individual's measure of strength or toughness (Ross and Schrader, 2021). Although this is a known fact by scientists in the academic settings, most of the population does not know. Many individuals tend to believe that PTSD only occurs in those who are mentally weaker because not everyone experiences PTSD after a traumatic event. As mentioned previously, many people questioned the likelihood of an individual developing PTSD among a group experiencing the same traumatic event. Those who are uninformed may believe that PTSD occurs to those who lack mental strength. In reality, all kinds of individuals have the ability to become a victim of PTSD regardless of their mental status. Any person at any time can experience symptoms of PTSD. PTSD symptoms are caused after trauma has been experienced by an individual, causing the body to go into a survival mode both mentally and physically, which then causes permanent changes to occur in the ways in which the brain functions (Howard, 2024).

IT IS ALL IN YOUR HEAD

PTSD does in fact exist, both in the academic and practical world. PTSD is a recognized mental health problem that has been around for hundreds of years. Nonetheless, it had been recognized throughout the years as various names, such as combat fatigue or shell shock (Ayaz, 2023). PTSD cannot be *all in your head* because unfortunately, in order to become a victim of PTSD, trauma has to occur. Trauma is an event that has caused the individual to fear for their life, see something horrible, or create feelings of helplessness. These strong emotions are caused by an event that results in changes to the brain structure, as well as the ways in which this individual now responds to their external environment (Forkus, 2023).

EVERYONE WHO HAS EXPERIENCED TRAUMA SHOULD BE AFFECTED

It is true that only a small percentage of individuals exposed to any kind of trauma actually experience symptoms of PTSD. This is due to the fact that every individual is different. Each individual that experiences trauma has his or her own set of risk factors for the possibility of developing PTSD (Ross and Schrader, 2021). These risk factors can include such things as the individual's genetics, past history of other traumas, as well as the degree or duration of their actual exposure to the traumatic event.

TREATMENT DOES NOT WORK

"Treatment does not work": This statement is false and derived from a lack of knowledge about academic workings. Several forms of therapy have proven to be effective in improving PTSD such as cognitive behavioral therapy (CBT), cognitive processing therapy, and desensitization (Murray, 2022). It has been a proven fact that there are many effective forms of treatment for PTSD. Each of these courses of treatment can be supported by not only written research, but also through implementation on those who are suffering from PTSD. Beyond therapy there are forms of medication that have shown improvement in individuals who are experiencing symptoms related to PTSD. It is important to understand that there is a possibility that a treatment will work for one individual but will not work for another. It takes some time to try various forms of treatment for one that will specifically help that individual.

ONLY SOLDIERS OR PEOPLE IN WAR ZONES GET PTSD

As stated before, anyone who sees or experiences a traumatic event has a possibility of developing PTSD. It does not matter where the traumatic event took place; whether it be in a backyard, at the mall, or in a military camp in Afghanistan, it is not significant. Soldiers are not the only victims of PTSD. It is a very common misunderstanding that began from its early stage of identification. Anyone can become a victim of PTSD (Ross and Schrader, 2021). It is simply a matter of chance and encountering an event that causes immense fear or a sense of losing control. These feelings can be triggered by a variety of situations such as violent crimes, sexual assaults, natural disasters, childhood neglect, first responders, and soldiers.

PEOPLE SHOULD BE ABLE TO MOVE ON AFTER TRAUMA

It is important to remember that PTSD is a medical condition; it is like any other disorder and there is no quick fix. It does, however, mean that these individuals suffering from PTSD have to learn how to live their life while dealing with their condition and trauma (Punski-Hoogervorst, 2022). This is similar to patients that have to learn to deal with cancer or bipolar disorder. The strong emotions that the individual feels during the traumatic event alter the way their brain functions. It is extremely difficult for the individual to go on as they normally would. They have to learn to adjust to a new way of living.

PEOPLE WITH PTSD CANNOT FUNCTION NORMALLY

Although PTSD can be associated with a few extreme symptoms, there is nothing that directly stops those affected from being able to live normal lives. Through the assistance of counseling, medicine, and family support, as well as friends, individuals are able to adjust to living with their symptoms. Individuals are recommended to seek treatment so that people are able to return to their regular routines prior to the trauma. Individuals diagnosed with PTSD can live happy lives, including holding a job and having healthy relationships (Ross and Schrader, 2021). The only thing that stands between an individual diagnosed with PTSD from living a fulfilling life is themself. It is up to the individual to make the decision to seek help.

PTSD ALWAYS HAPPENS DIRECTLY AFTER THE TRAUMA

The symptoms related to PTSD do not always occur immediately after trauma. For many individuals, it can take anywhere between one to three months for the more extreme symptoms to come into effect. There is even the chance that the symptoms won't surface beyond that amount of time. It is common for the symptoms of PTSD to come and go over a number of years. PTSD symptoms can slowly manifest themselves within the individual, until a strong memory or a stressful event brings forth a new strong symptom (Karstoft and Armour, 2022).

PTSD VICTIMS WILL NEVER GET BETTER

For many victims and as well as those close to the victim, they may feel that recovery is never possible. Fortunately, PTSD can be managed. In many cases, it can be defeated as long as the victim commits themselves to recovery. Every individual's recovery is dependent on the patient's sense of commitment and personal strength. Sometimes, it may seem that recovery is impossible and too monumental to overcome, but there are PTSD groups available to help victims (Bourassa, 2020). These support groups help to share success stories with others that may just now be experiencing PTSD symptoms. It is a way to build hope and strength for the newcomers.

PTSD SUFFERERS ARE UNSTABLE AND VIOLENT

Symptoms associated with PTSD vary depending on the individual—angry outbursts and violence do not always occur. Many believe that if the traumatic event was violent, then their symptoms will be very aggressive. PTSD is often associated with higher instances of aggression, many people with PTSD have not displayed aggressive behavior (Norman et al., n.d.). How a person reacts to the traumatic event, however, is dependent upon the individual's personal attributes and sensibilities and is irrelevant to the trauma itself. For example, if the traumatic event triggers an older violent memory, the individual is more likely to react aggressively. In most cases of PTSD, the severity of each of the symptoms will fluctuate and will almost never remain constant.

PTSD SUFFERERS AREN'T VICTIMS

There are people who are uninformed that believe PTSD sufferers are not victims but are actually people who seek attention from those around them. This is incorrect. PTSD sufferers are victims that have experienced a traumatic event that has altered their state of mind. These events are completely out of their own control. After a person becomes a victim of PTSD, they lack psychological ability to recover from the trauma by themselves. Trauma cannot simply be forgotten, and PTSD cannot be miraculously healed without external assistance. Individuals with PTSD need professional assistance to help them deal with the symptoms that affect their everyday lives.

REFERENCES

Ayaz, Y. "The Battle After the War: Portrayal of PTSD in Select Works of Modernist Fiction." *The Criterion: An International Journal in English* 14, no. V: 179–188, October 2023. https://www.the-criterion.com/V14/n5/WL01.pdf

Bourassa, K. J., D. J. Smolenski, A. Edwards-Stewart, S. B. Campbell, G. M. Reger, and A. M. Norr. "The Impact of Prolonged Exposure Therapy on Social Support and PTSD Symptoms." *Journal of Affective Disorders* 260: 410–417, January 2020. https://doi.org/10.1016/j.jad.2019.09.036

Forkus, S. R., A. M. Raudales, H. S. Rafiuddin, N. H. Weiss, B. A. Messman, and A. A. Contractor. "The Posttraumatic Stress Disorder (PTSD) Checklist for DSM–5: A Systematic Review of Existing Psychometric Evidence." *Clinical Psychology: Science and Practice* 30, no. 1: 110–121, March 2023. https://doi.org/10.1037/cps0000111

Howard, J., L. Lorenzo-Luaces, C. Lind, P. Lakhan, and L. A. Rutter. "Is a Criterion A Trauma Necessary to Elicit Posttraumatic Stress Symptoms?" *Journal of Psychiatric Research* 170, no. 2024: 58–64, February 2024. https://doi.org/10.1016/j.jpsychires.2023.12.008

Karstoft, K., and C. Armour. "What We Talk About When We Talk About Trauma: Content Overlap and Heterogeneity in the Assessment of Trauma Exposure." *Journal of Traumatic Stress* 36, no. 1: 71–82, September 25, 2022. https://doi.org/10.1002/jts.22880

Murray, H., N. Grey, E. Warnock-Parkes, A. Kerr, J. Wild, D. M. Clark, and A. Ehlers. "Ten Misconceptions About Trauma-Focused CBT for PTSD." *The Cognitive Behaviour Therapist* 15, no. 2022: e33, July 22, 2022. https://doi.org/10.1017/s1754470x22000307

Norman, S., E. B. Elbogen, and P. P. Schnurr. "Research Findings on PTSD and Violence." U.S. Department of Veterans Affairs, n.d. https://www.ptsd.va.gov/professional/treat/cooccurring/research_violence.asp#:~:text=Although%20PTSD%20is%20associated%20with%20increased%20risk%20of%20violence%2C%20most,diminishes%20(2%2C3)

Punski-Hoogervorst, J. L., A. Avital, and B. Engel-Yeger. "Challenges in Basic and Instrumental Activities of Daily Living Among Adults with Posttraumatic Stress Disorder: A Scoping Review." *Occupational Therapy in Mental Health* 39, no. 2: 184–210, July 8, 2022. https://doi.org/10.1080/0164212x.2022.2094523

Ross, A., and C. Schrader. "A Review of PTSD and Current Treatment Strategies." *The Journal of the Missouri State Medical Association* 118, no. 6: 546–551, December 2021. https://www.ncbi.nlm.nih.gov/pmc/articles/PMC8672952/pdf/ms118_p0546.pdf

CHAPTER 3

How to Assess

STRUCTURED INTERVIEWS

The most efficient method of assessing posttraumatic stress disorder survivors is through structured clinical interviews. It provides researchers with a thorough and standardized method of assessment for victims of PTSD. Through interviews, experts can follow with an in-depth exploration of what the victim is going through. It also gives the patient a safe space to share their thoughts and feelings about the traumatic event. It is important to recognize that as the patient reveals their experiences surrounding the trauma, there is the potential that it could reveal other traumatic events. This generally happens in the cases of sexual abuse victims. The more recent trauma brings light to past experiences that happened earlier in their lives. These clinical interviews are a standardized method for identifying the symptoms of PTSD.

STRUCTURED CLINICAL INTERVIEW

A structured clinical interview for the *DSM-V* (SCID-5) requires that a qualified social worker ask specific and direct questions about the client's symptoms. The SCID-5 has a PTSD section that has been shown to provide invaluable measurements that help identify the various aspects of PTSD being experienced by the patient ("The Structured Clinical Interview for DSM-5," n.d.).

PTSD SYMPTOM SCALE INTERVIEW (PSS-I AND PSS-I-5)

The PTSD Symptom Scale Interview (PSS-I and PSS-I-5) is composed of 17 *DSM-5* related items. The questions directed to the patient attempt to discover the individual's traumatic experiences and assess whether the various symptoms of the mental disorder being experienced by the patient is a consequence of the trauma or not. During this interview, people will select a single traumatic experience that is affecting them most and will answer the questions for experiences with this trauma over the previous two weeks. This is roughly a twenty-minute process of answering questions with no follow-ups ("PTSD Assessment Instruments," n.d.).

CLINICIAN-ADMINISTERED PTSD SCALE FOR DSM-5 (CAPS-5)

In addition to previously mentioned interviews and questionnaires, there is also a Clinician-Administered PTSD Scale for *DSM-5* (CAPS-5) that is administered at the same time as the others. This test measures the current status of the PTSD victim and the frequency and intensity of the distress associated with PTSD. For example, it measures the frequency of dreams related to traumatic events. CAPS-5 is a thirty-item structure interview that corresponds to the *DSM-5*'s criteria for PTSD and is said to be the highest rated test by psychologists assessing PTSD. CAPS-5 is very useful when diagnosing PTSD, as it can be used to make a current diagnosis of PTSD, create a lifetime diagnosis, and assess symptoms occurring as recently as one week. It is used for testing symptoms of PTSD, but also incorporates questions on how the PTSD victim is affected in social, occupational, and functional aspects of their lives. In addition, it compares the initial baseline test with a later administration of the CAPS-5 test to see if there have been any improvements in the patient's condition. The CAPS-5 has been created so that clinicians and clinical researchers can effectively oversee the test. The entire interview takes around forty-five–sixty minutes to administer ("PTSD Assessment Instruments," n.d.). Although, it is up to the clinician giving the test to decide on which parts of the test should be administered to the patient.

CLINICIAN-ADMINISTERED PTSD SCALE FOR CHILDREN AND ADOLESCENTS

Psychologists adapted the CAPS-5 to create the Clinician-Administered PTSD Scale for *DSM-5* – Child/Adolescent (CAPS-CA-5). CAPS-CA-5 is used to test for PTSD among children and adolescents from age 7 and up. This test consists of 20 *DSM-5* PTSD symptoms that were shown to be in association with a formal diagnosis of other PTSD victims. The test consists of the clinician asking the patient to rate the frequency and intensity of the twenty symptoms. CAPS-CA-5 is essential when diagnosing PTSD in children because it is extremely helpful in evaluating the impact the symptoms have on the child. The test analyzes the effects of the child's social, occupational, developmental functioning, subjective distress, global severity, and reaffirms the validity of this test. In general, CAPS-CA-5 helps create a lifelong timeline of PTSD ("Clinician-Administered PTSD Scale for DSM-5," n.d.).

SELF-REPORTS

This is an extremely important method of evaluation for assessing PTSD. Self-Report Instruments include the Davidson Trauma Scale (DTS), the Impact of Event Scale—Revised (IES-R), the Mississippi Scale for Combat-related PTSD (MISS or M-PTSD), the Modified PTSD Symptom Scale (MPSS-SR), the PTSD Checklist for *DSM-5* (PCL-5), the PTSD Symptom Scale Self-Report Version (PSS-SR), and the Short PTSD Rating Interview (SPRINT) ("PTSD Assessment Instruments," n.d.). These assessments allow the patient to give a personal analysis of what they are experiencing.

PTSD CHECKLIST FOR DSM-5 (PCL-5)

The PTSD Checklist for *DSM-5* (PCL-5) is a popular self-report method that consists of a twenty-item list that measures the *DSM-5* symptoms of PTSD. There are a variety of purposes for giving the PCL-5. This checklist helps to screen individuals for PTSD, test the diagnosis of PTSD, and to monitor the changes to the PTSD symptoms during and after the treatment. There are also three different versions of the PCL: military, civilian, and specific. PCL-M is used for military personnel and focuses on symptoms that are of consequence to military-related stress and experiences. It is given to active members of the service, as well as veterans. PCL-C includes questions that seek to discover the civilian's symptoms in relation to stressful life experiences. The PCL-C version is extremely important as it can be used with any population category. Its versatility allows clinicians to analyze a more general audience and a wider range of experiences and traumas. The final PTSD self-report test is known as PCL-S and is used for specific instances and to ask about symptoms that are in specific relation to a stressful experience. In addition to this, a patient may also be asked to complete the PCL-C corresponding to the specific events ("Posttraumatic Stress Disorder Checklist for the *DSM-5* [PCL-5]," n.d.). The PCL is a self-report measure, only the victim of PTSD can complete it. The test takes only five–ten minutes and can be completed in a waiting room before an actual clinical structured interview with the patient.

DISTRESSING EVENT QUESTIONNAIRE

The Distressing Events Questionnaire (DEQ) is another self-report method. The test consists of thirty-eight items that have been divided into four parts that assess the criteria from *DSM* on PTSD. Part one of the DEQ asks the patients to indicate the specific event that caused them the most distress within the past month. Then, they are to rate the degree to which they experienced each of the seventeen associated symptoms to PTSD. Each of the items are scored on a systematic rating scale that goes from 0 (absent) to 4 (extreme or severe degree). Part two asks the victim to state if they have experienced any of their symptoms for longer than thirty days. If the victims have, then they are to state when the symptoms began. Part three's questions require "yes" or "no" responses to assess symptoms of PTSD such as intense fear, helplessness, and horror. Part four analyzes more of the day-to-day areas of the patient's functioning such as social life, work life, and overall general satisfaction with life. Each of these items is once again scored on a four-point systematic grading scale, 0 (none) to 4 (extreme or severe degree). DEQ is important because it can be used as a preliminary diagnosis of PTSD to establish a cutoff score of the symptom's severity ("Distressing Event Questionnaire," n.d.).

CRITERIA FOR PTSD

When trying to understand PTSD through a psychological perspective, it is critical to gain further knowledge of how the *Diagnostic Statistical Manual* has qualified symptoms of PTSD. The *DSM-V* has divided the diagnostic criteria into eight groups (*DSM-V*, 2022).

"A" is the stressor criterion. It specifies a person that has experienced or been exposed to a catastrophic event that involved actual or threatened death, injury, sexual violence, or a threat to the physical integrity of him or herself. During this criterion, the survivor's subjective response is marked by intense fear, helplessness, or horror.

"B" is the intrusive recollection criterion. The symptoms for this section are very distinct and can remain for varying amounts of time. These symptoms are psychological experiences that cause the victims strong waves of panic, terror, dread, grief, and despair. These feelings are evident in the victim's daytime fantasies, nightmares, and PTSD flashbacks to the moment of trauma.

"C" is the avoidant or numbing criterion. Avoidance behavior consists of actions that reflect behavioral, cognitive, or emotional strategies that victims use to try to reduce their exposure to trauma-related stimuli. Patients also use these same strategies to attempt to minimize their psychological responses to the stimuli. Behavior strategies consist of trying to physically avoid any situation where the victim is exposed to trauma-related stimuli. In some of the more extreme cases, individuals shut themselves inside spaces to avoid contact with triggers that stimulate their psychological responses; this is called psychic numbing. Through this process, the individuals keep themselves emotionally intact, but it also makes it extremely difficult for these same individuals to create interpersonal relationships with others.

"D," involves negative changes in cognitive function and mood which occur either after a traumatic event or worsen after a traumatic event. Some people may experience a loss of memory associated with the traumatic event, consistent self-hate, consistent self-blame, severe depression, lack of interest in hobbies or social activities, feelings of loneliness or detachment, and/or a strong inability to experience good emotions.

"E," the fifth criterion, involves a state of hyperarousal, which closely resembles other mental health concerns, such as panic and anxiety disorders. While some victims of PTSD may suffer from anxiety and distress, it is more common for them to become hypervigilant; they become extremely anxious, paranoid, and always on alert. Hypervigilance is probably one of the most frequently occurring symptoms of PTSD.

"F," the duration criterion, establishes how long symptoms must persist before qualifying as a PTSD diagnosis. In the third version of the *DSM*, the symptoms had to persist for six months, but as of the fourth edition the period has been shortened to one month.

"G," the seventh criterion, is functional significance. It identifies the symptoms that have an influence on either the PTSD victim's social or occupational life. These influences are usually severe and extreme.

"H," the final criterion, is a note that the criterions are not induced by any type of substance such as drugs, or alcohol, or other medical conditions.

REFERENCES

"Clinician-Administered PTSD Scale for DSM-5 - Child/Adolescent Version (CAPS-CA-5)." PTSD: National Center for PTSD, n.d. https://www.ptsd.va.gov/professional/assessment/child/caps-ca.asp

Diagnostic and Statistical Manual of Mental Disorders: DSM-5-TR (DSM-V). American Psychiatric Association Publishing, 2022.

"Distressing Event Questionnaire." APA PsychNet, n.d. https://psycnet.apa.org/doiLanding?doi=10.1037%2Ft02170-000

"Posttraumatic Stress Disorder Checklist for the DSM-5 (PCL-5)." Traumadissociation.com, n.d. http://traumadissociation.com/pcl5-ptsd

"PTSD Assessment Instruments." American Psychological Association, n.d. https://www.apa.org/ptsd-guideline/assessment

"The Structured Clinical Interview for DSM-5®." American Psychiatric Association, n.d. https://www.appi.org/products/structured-clinical-interview-for-dsm-5-scid-5

4

HOW THE BRAIN COPES WITH
DIFFERENT TYPES OF TRAUMA

While everyone experiences stress throughout their daily lives, when one feels a strong emotional response to an extremely stressful or disturbing event, they undergo a traumatic experience. This experience is the body's natural response to threat. The response can vary in severity and impact, depending on the type and nature of the traumatic events. Trauma, along with adverse childhood experiences and chronic stress, is often the root cause of many chronic health disorders, such as anxiety, depression, posttraumatic stress disorder (PTSD), and addiction (Nelson et al., 2020). Although these nervous system dysfunctions do not always directly follow trauma, knowing the signs, symptoms, and effects of trauma is vital for prevention and treatment of its resulting disorders, especially since studies suggest that over 75% of Canadians have been exposed to at least one traumatic event in their lifetime (McCall and Watson, 2022). This chapter briefly introduces the types of traumas, outlines the functions and divisions of the nervous system, details an explanation of the brain's response to trauma, and discusses some PTSD treatment options.

By definition, trauma is an overall experience, not an event (Leonard, 2020). The American Psychological Association describes trauma as an emotional response to experiencing or witnessing events that involve actual or threatened death, serious injury, or sexual violence (Leonard, 2020). There are different types of traumas, including acute, chronic, and complex trauma. Acute trauma results from a single stressful event, while chronic trauma results from repeated exposure to a stressful event. Complex trauma occurs when one encounters multiple different traumatic events. One can also develop secondary trauma, which is a response to someone else's traumatic experiences. Accidents, assaults, abuse, disasters, rape, neglect, lack of safety, living in a war zone, and childhood medical procedures are all examples of traumatic situations that trigger a strong reaction from the body's nervous system (Leonard, 2020). Some studies also suggest that trauma can be passed down genetically through epigenetic mechanisms like DNA methylation (Fraga and Erdelyi, 2022).

Trauma is a normal emotional and physical reaction of the nervous system to an abnormal event. The nervous system's complex network of nerves and specialized cells (neurons) communicate to transmit signals throughout the body, therefore maintaining homeostasis and keeping one safe, especially during a threatening event. Whether this event is perceived as physically, mentally, or emotionally dangerous, the body generally has the same response because the same parts of the nervous system are activated. The two main divisions of the nervous system are the central nervous system (CNS), which consists of the brain and spinal cord, and the peripheral nervous system (PNS), which consists of everything else that extends to the rest of the body. The PNS has two divisions as well—the autonomic nervous system (ANS) and the somatic nervous system (SNS). The ANS controls the self-regulated action of internal organs and glands, while the SNS controls muscles and movement (Reebs, 2021). When dealing with trauma, the ANS is most important. This is because the ANS is further divided into sympathetic and parasympathetic systems. The sympathetic division, also known as the fight-or-flight division, prepares the body for stressful and emergency situations. It provides the body with a burst of energy so that it can respond to perceived physical, mental, or emotional dangers. The parasympathetic division of the nervous system controls bodily processes during ordinary situations by conserving and restoring energy. It is often called the "rest and digest" system, as it also calms the body down after the danger has passed (Reebs, 2021).

The three main chemical messengers (neurotransmitters) that communicate within the ANS are acetylcholine, epinephrine (also known as adrenaline), and norepinephrine (noradrenaline). As part of neurons, cholinergic nerve fibers secrete acetylcholine and adrenergic nerve fibers secrete epinephrine and norepinephrine (Hakala et al., 2021). Generally, acetylcholine has parasympathetic (inhibiting) effects and norepinephrine has sympathetic (stimulating) effects (Coon, 2023). Acetylcholine, however, has some sympathetic effects, as it sometimes stimulates sweating (Coon, 2023). A regulated nervous system uses the aforementioned neurotransmitters to experience stress and to also calm itself down throughout the course of a given day. For example, when one rushes to achieve an important time-sensitive task, the SNS division of their ANS is automatically activated. Once the task is completed in time, the body relaxes and energy is restored as the PNS division maintains balance in the body ("Autonomic Nervous System," 2022).

Trauma pushes the activation of the nervous system beyond its ability to self-regulate. When an extremely stressful experience, like a car accident, a destructive tsunami, or a serious injury, overworks the sympathetic nervous system beyond its normal ability, the system can become stuck in an active mode, even after the traumatic event has passed (Maynard, 2020). In the case of chronic trauma, the event reoccurs and often has worse consequences for the nervous system. This constant overstimulation of the body's fight-or-flight response causes anxiety, anger, hyperactivity, panic, and restlessness; the body becomes ready to fight or flee at all times because it still feels the need to protect itself (Maynard, 2020). It is not able to differentiate between its unsafe past and its safe present. It has to be retrained with the help of professionals and trusted individuals who are able to provide opportunities for cognitive behavioral therapy (CBT), desensitization, coregulation, sensorimotor therapy, and more to bring the nervous system back to normal and make it more flexible and resilient (Leonard, 2020). Some sympathetic nervous systems will fall below the normal range of activity and become stuck in an inactive mode instead (Maynard, 2020). This causes symptoms of fatigue, depression, disconnection, and lethargy. Systems can get stuck in one state for prolonged periods of time, or they can vary between the two modes.

Depending on the duration and severity of the systems' responses, illnesses can develop. For instance, doctors start considering PTSD as a diagnosis if the symptoms of ANS overstimulation exceed one month

("Traumatic Stress Section," n.d.). These symptoms can include recurrent unwanted memories and flashbacks of the traumatic event, upsetting dreams or nightmares about the event, severe emotional distress or physical reactions to something that reminds the patient of the traumatic event, and more (Mann and Marwaha, 2023). If the symptoms persist beyond three months, the individual is considered to have chronic PTSD. Moreover, there are several risk factors that also help predict the onset of PTSD. An article written in 2021 by doctors Angelica Staniloiu and Anthony Feinstein on the Canadian Encyclopedia states that being female, being younger at the time of the trauma exposure, having a history of previous trauma (especially during childhood), having a past/family psychiatric history, having lower education, and a lower intelligence quotient all increase one's risk of developing PTSD after trauma exposure. Staniloiu and Feinstein suggest that social support before and after the traumatic event is a key protective factor against the development of PTSD. They also mention that certain gene variants may protect an individual after exposure to traumatic events, while others may confer a vulnerability to developing PTSD (Staniloiu and Feinstein, 2021). The genetic composition of PTSD however is still not fully understood and is currently being studied by large-scale genome-wide association studies (GWAS). The nature of the trauma and one's coping strategies after it are two factors that also contribute to the development of PTSD. Acts of violence, sexual assault in particular, are especially traumatic, and insufficient or inappropriate coping strategies after trauma increase the risk of ANS overstimulation for prolonged periods of time (Staniloiu and Feinstein, 2021).

Aside from PTSD, the Canadian Psychological Association mentions that major depression is also a common problem following exposure to trauma. Major depression is more than your typical sadness. It involves a continuous feeling of deep sadness, no interest in normal daily routines, and more. It has been calculated that roughly half of the people who suffer with PTSD also suffer from depression, and that is not the only comorbid condition with PTSD. Comorbidities span from panic disorders to substance abuse disorders, as well as a myriad of physical health issues ("Traumatic Stress Section," n.d.). These abnormalities can be avoided by increasing one's window of tolerance, seeking safe relationships, finding a therapist, and practicing mindful breathing, which will be discussed in further detail at the end of this chapter.

More specifically, the stress response of the body starts in the brain. The amygdala, an area of the brain that contributes to emotional processing, plays a major role in the response to stressful events. It sends a distress signal to the hypothalamus, which functions like a command center and communicates with the rest of the body so that one has the energy to fight or flee ("Understanding the Stress Response," 2020). This area of the brain controls involuntary body functions such as breathing, blood pressure, heartbeat, and the dilation or constriction of key blood vessels and small airways in the lungs called bronchioles. After the amygdala sends a distress signal, the hypothalamus activates the sympathetic nervous system by sending signals through the autonomic nerves to the adrenal glands ("Understanding the Stress Response," 2020). These glands respond by pumping epinephrine into the bloodstream. As epinephrine circulates through the body, it causes many physiological changes, including a faster heartbeat than normal, higher blood pressure, and more blood being pushed to the muscles, heart, and other vital organs. The amygdala and the hypothalamus are both part of a group of structures in the brain that form the limbic system. One of its major functions is to respond to emotional stimuli, making it vital for ANS and PNS regulation (Neurol, 2023). This system also includes the hippocampus, thalamus, and nucleus accumbens ("Trauma to the Brain," n.d.).

As epinephrine continues spreading throughout the body, the person facing trauma also starts to breathe more rapidly. Any small airways in their lungs open wide to help the lungs take in as much oxygen as possible with each breath. With an increased oxygen supply to the brain, the person becomes more alert and sight, hearing, and other senses become sharper. Epinephrine also triggers the release of blood sugar (glucose) and fats from temporary storage sites in the body. These nutrients flood into the bloodstream, supplying energy to all parts of the body ("Understanding the Stress Response," 2020).

All of these changes happen so quickly that people are not aware of them. In fact, the wiring is so efficient that the amygdala and hypothalamus start this even before the brain's visual centers have had a chance to fully process any dangerous event ("Understanding the Stress Response," 2020). This is why people reflexively remove their hand from a hot surface before they feel the actual heat. According to an article posted by Harvard Health Medical School, after the initial brain response including a surge of epinephrine begins to recede, the next part in the brain's response to stress is activated by the hypothalamus. This part is called the HPA axis. The components of the brain that work to achieve these responses include the hypothalamus, and the pituitary and adrenal glands ("Understanding the Stress Response," 2020). The article compares the sympathetic nervous system to a gas pedal in a car and the parasympathetic system to the brakes. The gas pedal in the car is likened to the flow of hormonal signals that the HPA axis requires in order to keep the sympathetic nervous system moving forward. After continued perceived threat the brain will release a corticotropin-releasing hormone (CRH), which triggers the release of adrenocorticotropic hormone (ACTH) once it reaches the pituitary gland. Cortisol is released by the adrenal glands which are triggered by the arrival of ACTH. The braking system works by lowering cortisol levels once the threat has passed and the parasympathetic nervous system can put the brakes on the initial stress response ("Understanding the Stress Response," 2020).

The stress response becomes harmful when the ANS constantly signals danger, even when one is safe. People often develop adaptive strategies like using drugs, alcohol, food, or work to bring temporary relief to the constant stress. This may also damage the PNS and prevent it from functioning optimally. After trauma, the brain becomes easily triggered by sensory input, as it starts reading normal circumstances as dangerous (Kearney and Lanius, 2022). For instance, seeing a red light starts to become an indication of a possible spark or danger. A barbecue no longer seems normal, but might seem more threatening, like an explosion. These instances of sensory overload can be misinterpreted, which causes the brain to lose its ability to differentiate between what is threatening and what is normal.

The prefrontal cortex in the front part of the brain is where one's consciousness processes information and makes meaning of language. When trauma occurs and one enters a fight-or-flight mode, the prefrontal cortex can enter a freeze state as well, which shuts it down (Maynard, 2020). As a result, the brain becomes disorganized and overwhelmed while the body goes into survival mode and shuts down the higher order reasoning and language structures of the brain (Maynard, 2020). After the event, the memory of the experience is not reliable because the hippocampus, which processes memories, is too busy encoding information during a traumatic event (Maynard, 2020). The physiological, psychological, and behavioral responses to trauma and PTSD are discussed in further detail in Chapter 8 of this book.

The treatment options for the abnormal conditions that result from trauma can vary. Some common approaches to trauma therapy include cognitive-behavioral therapy (CBT), psychodynamic therapy, sensorimotor therapy, eye movement and desensitization reprocessing (EMDR), and pharmacological treatment ("Trauma," n.d.). According to the Centre for Addiction and Mental Health, there is a great deal of benefit to be achieved from treatment plans that are informed by the trauma of the individual patient. This care involves using approaches that not only validate the patient, but that are also uniquely shaped to the individual experience a person is having with PTSD. The "trauma-informed" approach has a complex understanding of all potential symptoms of trauma and considered coping strategies for treating each type of response to traumatic events. This treatment method is entirely non-judgmental and focuses its understanding of how different people may have different mental or physical responses to any sort of overwhelming stressors ("Trauma," n.d.).

Traditional methods of treatment have attempted to access the rational part of the brain through talk therapy. Talking through an event was thought to help a person become desensitized to the emotional intensity of the event. This is generally aimed at helping the individual understand that the danger does not persist beyond the event itself. Although these methods helped, they did not address the physiological responses of the ANS that often remained even after talking through the trauma (Dennis, 2021). In the last two decades, brain scan technology has allowed researchers to gain insight into what happens to the brain and body when people talk about the trauma versus when people reexperience it. Researchers found that talk therapy attempts to engage the parts of the brain that are not active when remembering or re-experiencing trauma, which does not resolve people's hyperdistressed states (Dennis, 2021).

There have been many advancements in understanding how the brain works in conjunction with traumatic experiences. As such, psychiatrists and therapists should be acutely aware of how the brain responds to trauma in order to better help their patients learn about and understand their reactions to trauma. Knowing how the brain copes with trauma can give ideas and information for both understanding of the illness and treatment. Learning about the neurobiology of trauma involves learning about the ways in which brain chemistry is altered during a traumatic event ("Neurobiology of Trauma," n.d.). The human brain recircuits itself as a protective or coping mechanism which results in the aforementioned symptoms for PTSD. People relive traumatic events or experience hyperarousal because their brains are now hard-wired to avoid ever facing such trauma again.

Additionally, although traditional treatments for PTSD involve talk therapy and finding meaning in the traumatic event, newer treatment methods involving calming the arousal system within the brain might help to reduce the effects of PTSD significantly more than can be done through any sort of talking or reasoning. This kind of treatment is known as "bottom-up processing" (Cherry, 2023). This kind of treatment soothes and calms the body by avoiding trauma questions that can escalate distress and further imprint trauma into the limbic system. Eye movement desensitization and reprocessing (EMDR) is one treatment option that uses bilateral stimulation to activate both sides of the brain. Bilateral movement causes the traumatic memory that remains in the emotional part of the brain to integrate with the cognitive part of the brain (McClelland and Gilyard, 2019). This increases the ability of the prefrontal cortex to become more active and find the rationality of the traumatic event. Daniel Amen, a popular American psychiatrist and brain disorder specialist, has documented through his neuro-imaging studies that people experience calm reactions following EMDR treatment (Dennis, 2021).

Another form of treatment is sensorimotor therapy, which helps a person become more in tune with their mind and body to heal collectively. Rocking back and forth, meditating, breathing deeply, exercising, and praying can all stimulate the PNS and calm the limbic system structures in the brain. Some therapists recommend setting aside five minutes every day to be open to any thoughts, sensations, or feelings that are associated with the patient's trauma (Persichilli et al., 2022). Whenever painful internal feelings arise during the rest of the day, the patient can acknowledge the thoughts, feelings, or images and remind oneself that they can come back during the five minutes set aside for them. This helps some patients be more present and available throughout the day. Regardless of the method of treatment, however, therapists must be contacted for expert help when dealing with trauma and its effects, especially if the trauma is chronic.

Overall, healing from trauma is not an easy process. With time, the intensity of the emotional pain generally decreases because the brain, being geared for survival, eventually prioritizes new threats and information and directs one's attentional resources to what is potentially important (Persichilli et al., 2022). Avoidance behaviors, including ignoring the pain and trying to suppress it, tend to keep the emotional pain active at the front of the mind, which slows the healing process. Studies have shown a correlation between avoidance behaviors and the development of PTSD (Persichilli et al., 2022). The more one tries to avoid thinking about a traumatic event, the more likely one is to develop PTSD. Therefore, one must ensure that they receive adequate treatment after experiencing trauma to prevent the development of chronic conditions that become more difficult to treat over time.

REFERENCES

"Autonomic Nervous System." 2022. Cleveland Clinic. https://my. clevelandclinic.org/health/body/23273-autonomic-nervous-system

Cherry, K. "How Bottom-Up Processing Works." Verywell Mind, March 6, 2023. https://www.verywellmind.com/bottom-up-processing-and-perception-4584296

Coon, E. "Overview of the Autonomic Nervous System—Brain, Spinal Cord, and Nerve Disorders." Merck Manuals, July 2023. https://www.merckmanuals.com/en-ca/home/brain,-spinal-cord,-and-nerve-disorders/autonomic-nervous-system-disorders/overview-of-the-autonomic-nervous-system

Dennis, J. "You Can't Logic Out of Trauma—Mindful Counseling." Mindful Counseling, 2021. https://mindfulcounselingutah.com/blog/youcantlogicoutoftrauma

Fraga, J., and K. M. Erdelyi. "Can Trauma Be Passed Down from One Generation to the Next?" Psycom.net, August 31, 2022. https://www.psycom.net/trauma/epigenetics-trauma

Hakala, S. M., M-P. Meurville, M. Stumpe, and A. C. LeBoeuf. "Biomarkers in a Socially Exchanged Fluid Reflect Colony Maturity, Behavior, and Distributed Metabolism." *eLife* 10, November 2, 2021. https://doi.org/10.7554/elife.74005

Kearney, B. E., and R. A. Lanius. "The Brain-Body Disconnect: A Somatic Sensory Basis for Trauma-Related Disorders." *Frontiers* 16, October 14, 2022. https://www.frontiersin.org/journals/neuroscience/articles/10.3389/fnins.2022.1015749/full

Leonard, J. "What Is Trauma? Types, Symptoms, and Treatments." *Medical News Today*, June 3, 2020. https://www.medicalnewstoday.com/articles/trauma

Mann, S. K., and R. Marwaha. "Posttraumatic Stress Disorder." StatPearls [Internet], January 30, 2023. https://www.ncbi.nlm.nih.gov/books/NBK559129/

Maynard, E. "Correlation Between Structures of the Brain Function and PTSD." Verywell Mind, February 13, 2020. https://www.verywellmind.com/what-exactly-does-ptsd-do-to-the-brain-2797210

McCall, C. A., and N. F. Watson. "A Narrative Review of the Association between Post-Traumatic Stress Disorder and Obstructive Sleep Apnea." *Journal of Clinical Medicine*, 11, no. 2, January 14, 2022. https://doi.org/doi: 10.3390/jcm11020415

McClelland, D., and C. Gilyard. "Calming Trauma—How Understanding the Brain Can Help." Phoenix Society for Burn Survivors, 2019. https://www.phoenix-society.org/resources/calming-trauma

Nelson, C. A., R. D. Scott, Z. A. Bhutta, N. B. Harris, A. Danese, and M. Samara. "Adversity in Childhood is Linked to Mental and Physical Health Throughout Life." *thebmj*, 371: m3048, October 28, 2020. https://www.bmj.com/content/371/bmj.m3048

"Neurobiology of Trauma." Assault Survivors Advocacy Program, n.d. https://unco.edu/assault-survivors-advocacy-program/learn_more/neurobiology_of_trauma.aspx

Persichilli, G., J. Grifoni, M. Pagani, M. Bertoli, E. Gianni, T. L'Abbate, L. Cerniglia, G. Bevacqua, L. Paulon, and F. Tecchio. "Sensorimotor Interaction Against Trauma." *Frontiers in Neuroscience* 16, June 14, 2022. https://doi.org/10.3389/fnins.2022.913410

Reebs, B. "Chronic Disease Archives." Modern Vital, June 28, 2021. https://www.drreebs.com/category/chronic-disease/

Staniloiu, A., and A. Feinstein. "Post-Traumatic Stress Disorder (PTSD) in Canada." *The Canadian Encyclopedia*, 2017. https://www.thecanadianencyclopedia.ca/en/article/post-traumatic-stress-disorder-ptsd-in-canada

"Trauma." Center for Addiction and Mental Health, n.d. https://www.camh.ca/en/health-info/ mental-illness-and-addiction-index/trauma

"Traumatic Stress Section: Facts About Traumatic Stress and PTSD." Canadian Psychological Association, n.d. https://cpa.ca/sections/traumaticstress/simplefacts/

"Trauma to the Brain—The Limbic System." Pivotal Education, September 28, 2017. https://pivotaleducation.com/hidden-trainer-area/ training-online-resources/trauma-brain-limbic-system/

"Understanding the Stress Response." Harvard Health, July 6, 2020. https://www.health.harvard.edu/staying-healthy/understanding-the-stress-response#:~:text=It%20triggers%20the%20fight%2Dor,after%20the%20danger%20has%20passed

CHAPTER 5

POTENTIAL CAUSES OF *PTSD*

Psychotraumatology is the study of psychological trauma and treatment, prevention, and people's reactions associated with traumatic situations. It was also understood that the brain copes differently with the different types of traumas. How are all these topics related to PTSD? PTSD, which stands for posttraumatic stress disorder, is a chronic physiological disorder which occurs after one's exposure to a traumatic event, 7%–8% of the US population suffering from PTSD at some point in their lives ("How Common Is PTSD?," n.d.). In a given year, about eight million US adults suffer from PTSD. Individuals who suffer from PTSD are only a small proportion of people who go through a trauma, with women being more likely to develop PTSD at some point in their lives compared to men with the relative ratio being 10%-4% ("How Common Is PTSD?," n.d.). So, the question that is often asked is: why do some people develop PTSD while others do not? Therefore, in this chapter the question "What are the potential causes of PTSD?" will be explored.

As discussed earlier, PTSD is a mental health problem that is developed after people experience or witness a traumatic or a life-threatening situation such as a natural disaster, a car accident, sexual assault, and so on ("Posttraumatic Stress Disorder [PTSD]," 2022). It is a disorder that is listed in the *Diagnostic and Statistical Manual of Mental Disorder (DSM)*. According to the *DSM*, the traumatic event must include exposure to actual or threatened death, serious injury, or learning about a trauma that occurred to an extremely close family member or friend

(*DSM-V*, 2022). The term *exposure* is defined as directly experiencing or witnessing the traumatic event or learning that a traumatic event has occurred to their family members or friends, or through exposure to television, movies, pictures, or any other electronic medium ("What Is Considered a Traumatic Experience?" 2020).

In normal situations when one experiences a stressful event, their nervous system switches from a normal nonpanic mode to panic mode which reacts with a fight-or-flight response. Once the threat or danger has passed, however, the nervous system calms down and shifts back to the nonpanic mode. On the other hand, individuals who suffer from PTSD have their nervous system stuck in the fight or flight zone even after the danger or the threat has passed. Their nervous system is unable to return to the normal state of balance, hence, they are unable to move on from the event.

In terms of what potentially causes PTSD, the exact mechanisms that lead to the development of PTSD have not yet been fully discovered. Researchers however generally believe that PTSD is not caused by a single factor. In fact, the development of PTSD is a result of various factors that work together alongside or even prior to the traumatic event, commonly cited causes of PTSD include risk factors, genetics, neurobiology and the brain structures, environmental factors, and psychological factors ("PTSD: Statistics, Causes, Signs & Symptoms," 2021).

RISK FACTORS

Although trauma is a huge factor that results in the development of PTSD, the presentation of the development of PTSD has also shown to be affected by a number of individual and societal pretrauma risk factors. First of all, women are four times more likely than men to develop PTSD after exposure to a traumatic event (Sareen, 2022). Moreover, research suggests that the period of the traumatic event and an increased duration of exposure to a traumatic event is associated with higher risks of the development of PTSD (Sareen, 2022). Additionally, social support is one of the risk factors that can impact the potential development of PTSD, with little to no social support after a traumatic event being positively associated with the development of PTSD ("Posttraumatic Stress Disorder (PTSD)" 2022).

GENETICS

Research has shown that just like other psychiatric disorders, PTSD also has a huge genetic component. Almost 30% of PTSD cases can be explained by genetics alone ("Posttraumatic Stress Disorder," n.d.). This was also supported in a naturalistic study conducted to understand the heart rate reactions to PTSD. In this study, heart rate data from veterans diagnosed with PTSD was investigated to understand the various factors on heart rate. Of the ninety-nine veterans with PTSD, ninety-one participants reported at least one hyperarousal event, as demographic information was complete for thirty-eight participants, it was found that factors including smoking, sleeping, gender, and medication were strongly associated with PTSD symptoms (Sadeghi and Sasangohar, 2021). Other research has also shown that an abnormally large cavum septum pellucidum is associated with abnormal limbic system development serving as a risk factor for chronic PTSD, while smaller hippocampal volumes have also been correlated with PTSD (Ben-Zion et al., 2020). It is found that smaller hippocampal volume has adverse effects on stress hormones on the brain which results in extreme stress therefore smaller hippocampal volumes are also a risk factor for chronic PTSD (Ben-Zion et al., 2020). Therefore, the results of Roger and his colleagues' study support that genetics and family vulnerability factors play a huge role in the development of chronic PTSD upon the exposure of a traumatic event. This also suggests that the unexposed cotwins of combat veterans with PTSD are at high risk of developing PTSD in the future after encountering a traumatic event.

NEUROBIOLOGY AND THE BRAIN STRUCTURE

There are many biological abnormalities observed in patients suffering from PTSD. These abnormalities result in the dysregulation of multiple stress mediated systems within the PTSD patients. Pathophysiological perturbations occur due to genetics, epigenetics, as well as the experiential predisposition and exposure to the trauma, patients with PTSD also tend to lack the baseline cortisol at the time of psychological trauma (Engel et al., 2023). This may be the reason behind the over activation of the CRH-Ne Cascade which results in a prolonged and enhanced stress response, thus, this enhanced stress response may be elevated due to inadequate regulatory effects of the neurotransmitters gaba, serotonin, and MPY (Engel et al., 2023). Lastly, in terms of brain structures, a smaller hippocampus, increased activity in the amygdala, and decreased activity and volume of PFC, ACC, and OFC are all associated with PTSD (Kredlow et al., 2021).

PSYCHOLOGICAL FACTORS

Research has shown that people who are already predisposed to or suffer from other mental illnesses such as depression and anxiety are at a higher risk of developing PTSD (Sareen, 2022).

ENVIRONMENTAL FACTORS

PTSD has also been found to be positively correlated with previous exposure to trauma. Research has shown that those who have a previous history of trauma and stress are shown to be more likely to develop PTSD compared to those who were not exposed to trauma. A study done on Vietnam veterans showed that history of any previous traumatic exposure was associated with a greater risk of PTSD and that multiple previous traumatic events had a stronger effect than a single previous traumatic event (Volkers, 2022). The researchers also found that subjects who experienced multiple events of assaultive violence in their childhood were more likely to experience PTSD in adulthood (Volkers, 2022). Therefore, through the findings of this study, one can conclude d that previous exposure to trauma signals a greater risk of PTSD from subsequent trauma.

Additionally, early childhood neglectful experiences are also associated with greater risk of developing posttraumatic stress disorder. Childhood neglect is defined as an act performed by a parent or a caregiver which results in the child being deprived of their basic physical or psychological needs. Some of the most common types of childhood neglect include lack of supervision, failure to attend to psychological and emotional needs, failure to provide education, medical care, clothing, shelter, nourishment, as well as abandonment. These experiences are often very stressful, frightening, distressing, and often continue for a long period of time. This repeated experience of trauma early in development is known as complex trauma. Research suggests that repeated exposure to traumatic events in early development results in inhibiting the neural systems ability to return to a normal stress after encountering a stressful situation and activating the fight or flight response (Kearney and Lanius, 2022).

TRAUMATIC EXPERIENCES

One of the biggest and common factors that result in the development of PTSD is exposure to traumatic events. PTSD develops after the exposure to a potentially traumatizing event. In fact, according to the *Diagnostic and Statistical Manual of Mental Disorder*, the traumatic event must involve serious injury, sexual violence, or an actual or threatened act. There are many types of traumas that can result in a development of PTSD, for example, in men, witnessing another person being killed or badly injured, being in a life-threatening accident, and being threatened with a weapon are some of the most common traumatic events which can lead to PTSD (Sareen, 2022). Alternatively, among women; sexual abuse, experiencing a natural disaster, witnessing another person being killed or badly injured, and being in a life-threatening accident are the most common traumatic events (Sareen, 2022). Other recognized causes of PTSD include witnessing or experiencing serious physical, emotional, or sexual abuse, physical assault, sexual assault, drug addiction, natural or man-made disasters and even bullying by peers or mugging incidents (Sareen, 2022). In this chapter, some of the most common traumatic events will be discussed.

CAR ACCIDENTS

Car accidents are one of the most common types of life-threatening trauma experiences. Over 38,000 people died on US roads in 2023 while there are numerous lucky others who were involved in the dramatic crashes but were fortunate enough to survive. PTSD caused by motor vehicle accidents are among the leading causes of PTSD in America (Bieber, 2023; "What are the Causes of PTSD?" n.d.).

SEXUAL ASSAULT

Sexual assaults are one of the most frequent types of traumas experienced by women. It is a form of intense violation which brings a lot of emotional and physical trauma which can be very hard to cripple within a daily life. In most cases once one has been assaulted, the feeling of being attacked usually never truly goes away as there is no reset button in the body or the mind which can completely erase the event as if it had never occurred. The prevalence of PTSD in assault survivors is drastically higher than the national prevalence of the disorder itself. Nearly 50% of rape survivors developed PTSD at three months postrape and rape stigma was associated with an increase in PTSD symptoms at six months (Nöthling et al., 2022). An assault survivor may experience a dysregulation of the hypothalamic pituitary adrenal axis which is responsible for stress management, which may be the primary structural and functional abnormalities contributing to the PTSD symptoms. Although therapies are available to the survivors of assault, they are often inadequate or unwanted (Chivers-Wilson, 2020).

COMBAT

Combat is also one of the most common causes of PTSD among veterans and military personnel. Soldiers who were often called to serve are often exposed to long periods of the horror of war, death, food starvation, as well as extreme environments. Exposure to all these traumatic stressors often injure them for life through disorders such as PTSD which are often unseen. For example, for the US soldiers who returned from Iraq and were hospitalized for war-related injuries, there was a 4.2% prevalence rate of PTSD at one month postinjury and the prevalence rate of 12.2% at four months postinjury (Sareen, 2022). Moreover, the severity of physical problems after injury was also seen to be positively correlated with PTSD as soldiers who had high severity of physical problems a month after injury were at a higher risk of developing PTSD six months later compared to the soldiers with low physical problems severity. Additionally, half of the soldiers who had war related mild traumatic brain injury (TBI) met the criteria of PTSD (Sareen, 2022).

MASS CONFLICT AND DISPLACEMENT

A meta-analysis of 64,332 refugees found a 30.6% prevalence rate of PTSD among the refugees who experienced mass conflicts and displacement. It was reported that higher PTSD rates were associated with factors such as torture and cumulative exposure to dramatic events as well as assessed level of political terror (Sareen, 2022).

MEDICAL ILLNESS

Although medical illness might not seem to induce PTSD or related symptoms, research shows that serious physical illnesses are associated with PTSD. For example, an analysis of twenty-four observational studies showed that of the 2,383 patients who experienced an acute coronary syndrome, 12% experienced clinically significant levels of PTSD. The finding of this meta-analysis suggested that PTSD symptoms induced by acute coronary syndrome were moderately prevalent and associated with the recurrent cardiac events and increased risk of mortality. Additionally, there's growing literature which suggests that one in four cases of stroke or TIA may be associated with PTSD as stroke patients with symptoms of PTSD may have more anxiety about preventative medications and future stroke. Moreover, a 2008 systematic analysis of fifteen studies found that there is around a 20% prevalence of PTSD among the people who survived intensive care unit (ICU) hospitalization. Another study from 2015 showed that within one to six months of hospitalization, there was a 24% prevalence rate of PTSD symptoms among the patients and 22% prevalence after seven to twelve months. There are factors for PTSD associated with ICU such as early memories of frightening ICU experiences as well as the use of benzodiazepine. This shows that medical conditions which induce a lot of fear and anxiety are a potential threat to the patient which can induce PTSD (Sareen, 2022).

CHILDHOOD TRAUMA

Childhood is a critical period of time for both the physical and psychological development of an individual. Trauma in childhood can leave drastic effects on an individual and can take many forms from neglect to abuse (Pate, 2021). First of all, nonnormative life experiences such as repeated exposure to in-city violence have shown to induce posttraumatic stress disorder in children and adolescents. These situations do not include the child physically experiencing the trauma but witnessing trauma around them such as seeing someone being shot. Exposure to violence in childhood can significantly be related to PTSD and studies show that PTSD is only the first step of the psychopathological instance and that these children can later go on to develop depression and suicidal ideation (Pate, 2021).

Single exposures to no normative life events such as home fires or car crashes have also been seen to induce PTSD in children. House fire seems to have a greater impact as a child does not only face physical trauma but also loses the secure environment that they were used to. In a study, Greenberg and Kian found that 72% of the children who developed PTSD following a house fire continued to have posttraumatic symptomatology after nine months of the house fire (Pate, 2021). The study also found that older children are more prone to developing PTSD from house fires (Pate, 2021).

Normative life experiences such as loss of a parent can also cause posttraumatic stress disorder within children. According to the child bereavement study, 50% of the children aged three to six suffered from bereavement issues even after two years of their parents' death. Children with PTSD from the loss of a parent experience nightmares and activities that are symbolic of their trauma (Pate, 2021).

Another major childhood trauma that in most cases remains unreported is physical abuse. Children who are exposed to physical abuse tend to have more behavioral manifestations of PTSD. This may be due to the fact that children do not have the same capabilities as adults to express their feelings through emotions and words therefore they tend to use their behavior and reactions to express their distress (Pate, 2021).

Lastly, one of the most commonly reported and researched sources of PTSD in children is sexual abuse however research on this is limited due to the fact that children do not or are unable to disclose what occurred to them. In many cases the diagnosis of PTSD and sexually abused children is delayed due to the fact that the disclosure of the abuse is not disclosed until the child is at a much later stage of age. There are also gender differences in the prevalence of symptoms of PTSD after child abuse as generally the victims of child sexual abuse are often females and that boys are usually less likely to admit to sexual abuse. In fact, girls are two to six times more likely to develop PTSD when this initial source of disorder is sexual abuse (Pate, 2021).

Overall, the exact cause of PTSD is still not known. It is predicted that PTSD is caused by the combination of factors such as genetics, brain structures, the intensity of the trauma, and other risk factors.

REFERENCES

Ben-Zion, Z., M. Artzi, D. Niry, N. J. Keynan, Y. Zeevi, R. Admon, H. Sharon, et al. "Neuroanatomical Risk Factors for Posttraumatic Stress Disorder in Recent Trauma Survivors." *Biological Psychiatry. Cognitive Neuroscience and Neuroimaging* 5, no. 3: 411–419, March 5, 2020. https://www.ncbi.nlm.nih.gov/pmc/articles/PMC7064406/

Bieber, C. "Car Accident Statistics for 2023." Forbes, February 5, 2024. https://www.forbes.com/advisor/legal/car-accident-statistics/.

Chivers-Wilson, K. "Sexual Assault and Posttraumatic Stress Disorder: A Review of the Biological, Psychological, and Sociological Factors and Treatments." *Mcgill Journal of Medicine* 9, no. 2, 2020. https://doi.org/10.26443/mjm.v9i2.663

Diagnostic and Statistical Manual of Mental Disorders: DSM-5-TR (DSM-V). Washington, DC: American Psychiatric Association Publishing, 2022.

Engel, S., S. Laufer, H. Klusmann, L. Schulze, S. Schumacher, and C. Knaevelsrud. "Cortisol Response to Traumatic Stress to Predict PTSD Symptom Development—A Systematic Review and Meta-Analysis of Experimental Studies." *European Journal of Psychotraumatology* 14, no. 2, July 4, 2023. https://www.ncbi.nlm.nih.gov/pmc/articles/PMC10321212/#

"How Common Is PTSD in Adults?" U.S. Department of Veterans Affairs, n.d. https://www.ptsd.va.gov/understand/common/common_adults.asp

Kearney, B. E., and R. A. Lanius. "The Brain-Body Disconnect: A Somatic Sensory Basis for Trauma-Related Disorders." *Frontiers*, October 14, 2022. https://www.frontiersin.org/journals/neuroscience/articles/10.3389/fnins.2022.1015749/full

Kredlow, A. M., R. J. Fenster, E. S. Laurent, K. J. Ressler, and E. A. Phelps. "Prefrontal Cortex, Amygdala, and Threat Processing: Implications for PTSD." *Nature News*, September 20, 2021. https://www.nature.com/articles/s41386-021-01155-7

Nöthling, J., N. Abrahams, R. Jewkes, S. Mhlongo, C. Lombard, S. M. Hemmings, and S. Seedat. "Risk and Protective Factors Affecting the Symptom Trajectory of Posttraumatic Stress Disorder Post-Rape." *Journal of Affective Disorders* 309: 151–64, July 2022. https://doi.org/10.1016/j.jad.2022.04.032

Pate, K. M. "Understanding Post-Traumatic Stress Disorder in Children: A Comprehensive Review." *Inquiries Journal* 13, no. 02, 2021. http://www.inquiriesjournal.com/a?id=1871

"Posttraumatic Stress Disorder (PTSD)." Mayo Clinic, December 13, 2022. https://www.mayoclinic.org/diseases-conditions/posttraumatic-stress-disorder/symptoms-causes/syc-20355967

"Posttraumatic Stress Disorder" Psychiatry Neuroimaging Laboratory, n.d. http://pnl.bwh.harvard.edu/education/what-is/posttraumatic-stress- disorder/

"PTSD: Statistics, Causes, Signs & Symptoms." The Refuge, A Healing Place, 2021. https://www. therefuge-ahealingplace.com/ptsd-treatment/effects-symptoms- signs/

Sadeghi, M., F. Sasangohar, A. D. McDonald, and S. Hegde. "Understanding Heart Rate Reactions to Posttraumatic Stress Disorder (PTSD) Among Veterans: A Naturalistic Study." Human Factors: *The Journal of the Human Factors and Ergonomics Society* 64, no. 1: 173–87, July 22, 2021. https://doi. org/10.1177/00187208211034024

Sareen, J. "Posttraumatic Stress Disorder in Adults: Epidemiology, Pathophysiology, Clinical Features, Assessment, and Diagnosis." Www.uptodate.com, September 15, 2022, https://www. uptodate.com/contents/posttraumatic-stress-disorder-in-adults-epidemiology-pathophysiology-clinical-features-assessment-and-diagnosis

Volkers, Nancy. "Study Finds Ongoing Mental Health Concerns for Vietnam Veterans." Office of Research & Development, March 17, 2022. https://www.research.va.gov/currents/0322-Study-finds-ongoing-mental-health-concerns-for-Vietnam-Veterans.cfm

"What Are the Causes of PTSD?" Bridges to Recovery, n.d. https://www.bridgestorecovery.com/posttraumatic-   stress-disorder/what-are-the-causes-of-ptsd/

"What Is Considered a Traumatic Experience?" League of Minnesota Cities, September 25, 2020. https://www.lmc.org/ptsd-mental-health-toolkit/warning-signs-and-diagnoses/what-is-considered-a-traumatic-experience/

CHAPTER 6

THE DANGERS OF PTSD

PTSD, which stands for posttraumatic stress disorder is a mental disorder that develops due to a traumatic experience that leads to the buildup of immense stress and trauma in an individual's life (Matthews et al., 2022). PTSD tends to develop in those who have been subjected to high levels of stress, trauma, loss, or violence. PTSD has been impacting lives for centuries and the earliest records of this disorder can be found in cases of veterans who served in the world wars. Posttraumatic stress disorder has impacted people from around the globe and is not unique to a single culture or region. In Canada, there is an 8.8% prevalence rate for lifetime PTSD (Matthews et al., 2022). A study that did a meta-analysis of existing literature further found that 12.3%–14.3% of Canadian participants in various studies reported having experienced at least one traumatic event that was distressing enough to trigger PTSD (Matthews et al., 2022). The dangers of PTSD include its heavy impact on the daily lives and experiences of people, their interpersonal relationships, and how they cope with other stressful and challenging circumstances in their daily life. Furthermore, since PTSD is complex, so is the treatment. It may take some time for individuals to find the most suitable treatment for their traumatic experiences and to develop coping skills unlike their lifestyle. Although it is important to note that treatment, which includes either therapy, medication, or a combination of both, is extremely important for a healthy recovery and the lack of proper treatment can lead to more adverse effects of PTSD. PTSD may also lead to the development of other disorders such as depression and anxiety leading to high chances of comorbidity which makes PTSD a rather dangerous and serious mental health condition (Matthews et al., 2022). The dangers of PTSD are not just limited to mental health, but they have an impact on an individual's physical health as well (Sih et al., 2023). Those who are diagnosed with PTSD often have poor physical health including the risk of developing cardiorespiratory problems, musculoskeletal problems, gastrointestinal, and immunological disorders (Sih et al., 2023).

There are many adverse thoughts, feelings, and behaviors individuals with PTSD go through and these symptoms tend to persist for quite some time. They include intrusive thoughts that are usually involuntary and distressing that continue to reoccur and are followed by intense and long-lasting feelings of distress as well as physiological reactions which are the body's way of responding to distress (Sih et al., 2023). Another common behavior is avoidance. Usually, it is avoidance of distressing thoughts and feelings, especially those that remind an individual of their past traumatic experiences. People with PTSD also tend to avoid places, conversations, people, activities, objects, and situations that remind them of their past trauma (Sih et al., 2023). Lastly, PTSD has adverse effects on one's ability to regulate their emotional and cognitive abilities. They usually find themselves in forgetful situations, unable to remember important details, which usually happens due to the constant efforts to suppress unwanted memories. Unfortunately, in the process of doing so, they tend to erase or suppress some important parts of the past from their memory. People with PTSD, especially those whose trauma is associated with people in their life, develop a negative perception about life and people in general. They feel as if people close to them are untrustworthy and this life is meant to hurt them which makes them isolate themselves and avoid being around people. This leads to constant feelings of fear, anger, frustration, loneliness, guilt, and shame (Sih et al., 2023).

PATIENT EXPERIENCE WITH PTSD

A glimpse of what posttraumatic stress disorder looks and feels like for a victim is important to understand in order to improve mental health literacy and reduce the stigma. As an adaptive biological trait, there is a positive correlation between fear of danger and fear generalization toward similar but distinct stimuli (Sih et al., 2023). In sexual assault cases, victims require support from different resources like police, social workers, and counselors to develop the courage to face their assailant in court. The possibility of victims generalizing that fear and recalling the traumatic experience becomes much greater when victims are expected to attend court hearings. It can be an extremely challenging task to even decide to face an assailant in court, let alone develop the courage to actually attend the court hearing. Soon after a case is concluded and court hearings are completed, some victims might slide into a constant state of negativity and depression. The fear and recall are even greater when encountering their assailant. For such reasons, victims often experience comorbidity between different mental illnesses such as depression and general anxiety disorder. Victims may become easily distraught and unable to live independently for this reason (Sih et al., 2023). Such experiences further exacerbate and compound the likelihood of developing traumatic recall memories. In instances where fear generalization occurs, they may experience low affect and it takes a significant length of time for treatment to have notable impacts (Sih et al., 2023).

Other dangers of PTSD, in addition to avoiding situations that serve as a reminder of trauma, heightened fear, and depression, include sleeplessness, anxiety attacks, and self-destructive thoughts (Gutiérrez et al., 2023). Substance use as a means of coping with PTSD is a very common yet destructive approach. A common substance used for relief from PTSD symptoms is alcohol. Mixing alcohol or any other drug with PTSD however affects mental health worse since it does not reinforce healthy coping mechanisms. For example, when one experiences intrusive thoughts, if they develop healthy coping mechanisms, they may try to reflect or remind themselves that they are in a much better place now or that their past is not powerful enough to impact their future. Although, if drinking alcohol or consuming other drugs for PTSD symptom relief is used as a coping mechanism, then the individual may find themself in a much worse condition once the effect of the drugs start to decrease and they will start experiencing withdrawal symptoms which will put them in a much more vulnerable and negative state (Gutiérrez et al., 2023).

There are many different risk factors that make an individual either susceptible to developing PTSD or make their diagnosis of PTSD difficult to cope with (Manhapra et al., 2021). Factors that put an individual at a higher risk of experiencing a traumatic event are called pre trauma factors. These include gender, prior exposure to trauma, history of mental disorders, low IQ levels, personality issues, and genetics. Females are much more likely to be diagnosed with PTSD than males (Manhapra et al., 2021). An analysis of traumatic experiences showed that even when men and women went through similar traumatic situations, women were at a higher risk for developing PTSD after experiencing those circumstances.

An important point to note is that while gender has been associated with the risk of developing PTSD, the socioeconomic status, age, and race of an individual are not associated with the likelihood of them developing posttraumatic stress disorder. This emphasizes how PTSD can be diagnosed to anyone who goes through some sort of trauma, regardless of their age, race, and culture. Having a low IQ, head injury, or any other cognitive disability puts an individual at a greater risk of developing PTSD. This is the case because those with cognitive vulnerabilities may find it challenging to perceive traumatic or difficult situations. It makes it much more difficult for them to deal with their experiences and regulate their thoughts and emotions, thus putting them on an edge when it comes to PTSD. Index trauma refers to the main trauma or events which elicited symptoms of PTSD, so individuals who have experienced trauma or stressors before the index trauma are also at the greater risk of developing PTSD (Manhapra et al., 2021). The diagnosis of other mental health conditions such as anxiety disorders, depression, or schizophrenia makes it challenging to deal with stress and trauma. This explains why it is associated with higher risk of being diagnosed with PTSD in the time shortly after a traumatic event (Manhapra et al., 2021). Individuals who deal with personality issues such as neuroticism and who have personality traits that tend to make them an avoidant and isolated individual are linked to a greater chance of developing PTSD after a traumatic experience.

PTSD is a serious mental health condition and one of its most dangerous aspects is the fact that it not only impacts the victim alone but also eventually impacts the patient's relationship with other people

(Gutiérrez et al., 2023). Trauma factors are related to the actual traumatic experience which led to the development of PTSD. These factors include assaultive trauma, severe physical injury, the overall severity of the trauma, and having the fear of death (Manhapra et al., 2021). Posttraumatic factors that make it challenging for an individual to cope with their feelings and eventually develop PTSD include having low social support, increased financial stress, having to stay in intensive care units, constantly having a high heart rate, extensive pain, experiencing acupressure stress disorder, and expiring a disability due to the trauma (Manhapra et al., 2021).

PTSD is a serious mental health condition and one of its most dangerous aspects is the fact that it not only impacts the victim alone but also eventually impacts the patient's relationship with other people. When individuals with PTSD come in contact with objects, people, or situations that remind them of their last trauma, they feel as if they are reliving their traumatic experience all over again. This can turn on their fight or flight response and elicit feelings of hopelessness, anger, and fear. Such things are classified as triggers since they trigger an emotional and physiological response (Gutiérrez et al., 2023). PTSD can have an impact on pregnancy and mothering. Women who went through sexual abuse and neglect during their childhood years can feel extremely anxious or triggered when they themselves are becoming mothers. Furthermore, past experiences of a miscarriage, death of a child, stillbirth, or a traumatic birthing experience can lead to the development of symptoms of PTSD in pregnant mothers (Gutiérrez et al., 2023). Having PTSD as a pregnant woman can impact how the mother views the idea of having and raising a child and all her perceptions about herself as a mother. These thoughts and feelings can be anxious where a woman feels incapable of being a good mother due to her past experiences with neglect or it can also trigger feelings of anger and frustration toward the pregnancy if the mother had experienced a traumatic pregnancy in the past or if she is a victim of sexual assault (Gutiérrez et al., 2023). Unfortunately, the cycle of abuse, neglect, and trauma may be hard to break for people suffering from PTSD. Studies have shown that families continue to face abuse and neglect for generations (Gutiérrez et al., 2023). Mothers with PTSD are usually also suffering from major depressive disorder and have problems dealing with their emotions. This increases the likelihood of angry outbursts and a loss of self-control. Besides the person with PTSD, anger and low self-control can also have profound impacts on the mental well-being of children. The dangers of PTSD extend beyond patients and affect the lives of those around them (Gutiérrez et al., 2023).

Individuals diagnosed with PTSD have a difficult time maintaining their romantic relationships (Russin et al., 2023). Complex posttraumatic stress disorder is not found in the *Diagnostic Statistical Manual of Mental Disorders,* but it involves a related exposure to stressful events which is different from the general posttraumatic stress disorder that involves a single traumatic event (Russin et al., 2023). People who deal with PTSD, especially complex PTSD, have a difficult time forming intimate relationships that are healthy. Survivors of trauma have profound trust issues which are the root cause of instability in intimate relationships. Those who experience complex posttraumatic stress disorder may have been through ongoing trauma and neglect as a child which could have conditioned them to not trust even the people closest to them as they are reminded of painful and harmful memories. The trauma that arises is due to perceptions of betrayal by people who the victim trusted and confided in. Consequently, survivors develop self-defense mechanisms that can create an overgeneralization of perceived danger and coping strategies that result in greater solitude. In turn, these experiences exacerbate their mental illness symptoms, increase the likelihood of comorbid illnesses, and are erroneously used as justifications affirming their fears (Russin et al., 2023).

Another factor that makes intimacy and romantic relationships difficult are "flashbacks" experienced by the individual with PTSD. Flashbacks are not simply memories or a reminder from the past, but they work as though the individual is reliving a traumatic experience. There are three common types of flashbacks which cause extreme distress. There are emotional, visual, and somatic flashbacks (Russin et al., 2023). Emotional flashbacks tend to be the most damaging for the survivor. When in an intimate relationship, survivors may suddenly be reminded of a traumatic experience by the gesture of their partners even if that gesture had underlying good intentions. The gesture alone could cause emotional outbursts that not only affect the patient with PTSD, but also the other partner in the relationship (Russin et al., 2023). Patients who experience complex PTSD tend to be hypervigilant and remain extremely conscientious of their surroundings as their brains are wired to remain on the lookout for any risk or potential harm. People suffering complex PTSD are extremely sensitive to loud noises or footsteps, and even the slightest changes in their environment can cause them to hyperventilate or find themselves in a fight or flight response. A perpetual state of hypervigilance can be exhausting for survivors, so they often wish to spend time alone in comfort zones that are less likely to agitate their fight or flight responses. The isolation from others can often lead to a lack of intimacy and adventure in romantic relationships which can greatly impact how significant others may feel about their bond with them (Russin et al., 2023).

The most dangerous consequence of PTSD in terms of romantic relationships is when the survivor chooses the wrong romantic partner due to their PTSD. Survivors of childhood assault and neglect often search for a partner who will serve as their rescuer. Someone who will come into their life to help them heal, care for them, and save them from their trauma. Patients with PTSD feel hopeless as they search for their romantic partner because they hope to find someone who can help them recover from their past and give them the love and care that wasn't present in their life in the past. Humans, however, are likely to have the tendency to pick partners who mimic the adult role models they had in their lives as a child (Russin et al., 2020). As such, survivors of trauma will often pick partners that often cause additional harm (Russin et al., 2020). This is because the victim's trauma responses due to PTSD will make them look beyond their partner's potential flaws and red flags which would otherwise have been considered as drastic concerns by those that do not suffer from PTSD. Patients of PTSD are seeking love and validation which is why they overlook the warnings and commit to someone who can end up just as abusive and narcissistic to them, as the other people from their past (Russin et al., 2023).

REFERENCES

Gutiérrez H., L., P. C. Mesón, C. É. Gallardo, C. P. Puente, and D. M. Morales. "Mother-Child Bond Through Feeding: A Prospective Study Including Neuroticism, Pregnancy Worries and Post-Traumatic Symptomatology." *International Journal of Environmental Research and Public Health* 20, no. 3, February 1, 2023. https://doi:10.3390/ijerph20032115

Manhapra, A., E. A. Stefanovics, T. G. Rhee, and R. A. Rosenheck. "Association of Symptom Severity, Pain and Other Behavioral and Medical Comorbidities with Diverse Measures of Functioning Among Adults with Post-Traumatic Stress Disorder." *Journal of Psychiatric Research* 134: 113–120, February 1, 2021. https://doi:10.1016/j.jpsychires.2020.12.063

Matthews, L. R., L. E. Alden, S. Wagner, M. G. Carey, W. Corneil, T. Fyfe, C. Randall, et al. "Prevalence and Predictors of Posttraumatic Stress Disorder, Depression, and Anxiety in Personnel Working in Emergency Department Settings: A Systematic Review." *Journal of Emergency Medicine* (0736-4679) 62, no. 5: 617–35, May 2022. https://doi:10.1016/j.jemermed.2021.09.010

Russin, S. E., E. L. Tilstra-Ferrell, F. J. Griffith, and C. H. Stein. "Dating in the Wake of Trauma and Abuse: Relationship Experiences of Individuals with Posttraumatic Stress Disorder." *Journal of Aggression, Maltreatment & Trauma* 32, no. 5: 763–83, May 2023. https://doi:10.1080/10926771.2022.2112338

Sih, A., H. J. Chung, I. Neylan, C. Ortiz-Jimenez, O. Sakai, and R. Szeligowski. "Fear Generalization and Behavioral Responses to Multiple Dangers." *Trends in Ecology & Evolution* 38, no. 4: 369–80, April 2023. https://doi:10.1016/j.tree.2022.11.001

CHAPTER 7

DIFFERENT TYPES OF *PTSD*

What is posttraumatic stress disorder? It is a title that is quite self-explanatory. When an individual directly or indirectly experiences any traumatic events, it has the possibility of triggering negative physical and mental symptoms. After the individual has gone through this trauma, it interferes with their personal ability to cope with issues pertaining to their daily life. It is also important to note that the trauma does not only have to be caused by the death of an individual. PTSD can be induced by anything that evokes a sense of fear or any sort of intense emotion. In general, posttraumatic stress disorder (PTSD) refers to the psychological disorder that develops as a result of experiencing trauma from a stressor (Mayo Clinic Staff, 2022). Although all posttraumatic stress disorders generally fall under the same category of trauma-based disorders, there exists heterogeneity in the manifestation and prognosis across different cases. Thus, the definition and classification of PTSD can vary. Often, this aspect is based on a specific diagnostic framework and how it chooses to define and categorize a psychological disorder. This chapter will expand on how PTSD is divided into subtypes through different diagnostic frameworks. Additionally, it will also explore the recent and proposed subtypes of PTSD explored and defined by literature.

The brain is severely impacted after an individual experiences or witnesses a trauma. The brain reacts to the trauma by directing a message to the brain, telling it that the body is in a state of danger. This results in the body going into the fight-or-flight mode, a survival reaction. This is a primitive response by our bodies and is unconscious. It is a state that prepares the body to flee from harm or danger that is threatening your individual sense of survival. When an individual starts to experience this state of fight or flight, their body goes into a state of hyperarousal. In this state, adrenaline is released, the heart rate increases, pupils dilate, breathing rate increases, and the body begins to sweat profusely. These stages occur to prepare the body for an immediate threat. The body then winds down from the state of increased adrenaline and realizes that the threat has passed and can now return to its original state. Their breathing slows, heart rate steadies, sweating stops, and their pupils go back to their normal size ("Neurobiology of Trauma," n.d.). A PTSD victim experiences consistent and long-lasting periods of hyperarousal. The body's fight-or-flight response never shuts down, keeping their body in a state of intense hyperarousal. This not only causes physical strain on the body, but also causes the sufferer to experience significant distress and impact on their social, personal, and occupational life.

It is important to note that not everyone who experiences trauma is guaranteed to experience posttraumatic stress disorder. A person's past and the nature of the trauma play an essential role in whether they will suffer from PTSD or not. In the United States, 6% of the population will suffer from PTSD at some point in their life. In any given year, roughly 5% of American adults will have existing struggles with PTSD. In 2020, this translates to about 13 million Americans suffering with PTSD ("How Common Is PTSD in Adults?" n.d.). Although there has been research done on the genetic predisposition to PTSD, there is no confirmation of this theory. A lot of controversy rises around the issue of whether PTSD is due to nature or nurture. It is the question of whether or not individuals are genetically predisposed (nature) or if individuals are affected by experience and circumstance (nurture). In present society, our highest rates of PTSD occur in men and women who have been in war zones or those who were in motor-vehicle accidents ("How Common Is PTSD in Adults? N.d.). Although war and accidents have the highest rate of causing PTSD, there are other possibilities:

- natural disasters (floods, hurricanes, tornadoes, volcanic eruption)

- rape or sexual assault (as a child or adult)

- terrorist attacks (9/11)

- torture or optical imprisonment

- domestic violence

- carjacking

- robbery

To begin, even with heterogeneity in PTSD cases and experiences of patients, PTSD does not have any distinct or uniform subtypes. As mentioned, the subtypes that exist differ depending on what diagnostic criteria are employed. For example, at present, the *Diagnostic and Statistical Manual of Mental Disorders V (DSM-V)* and *International Classification of Diseases – 11th Revision (ICD-11)* are the most accepted frameworks that define PTSD (Bovin et al., 2021). Moreover, while sharing similarities, both of them are distinct in defining PTSD. While the *DSM* does not further categorize PTSD into types, the *ICD-11* distinguishes PTSD into further types. Moreover, the world health organization lists PTSD to be of two distinct types in the *ICD-11*. The first main type of posttraumatic stress disorder is PTSD while the second main type is C-PTSD or also known as complex posttraumatic stress disorder (Cloitre, 2020). The main reason behind this distinction is the experiences of the patients and treatment outcomes. While a lot of traumas may occur as a one-time occurrence, in some cases patients face chronic and recurring trauma. Not only does this have an impact on symptomatology but also on treatment outcomes. Therefore, the *ICD-11* distinguishes complex PTSD from standard PTSD to define the cases that are not completely explained but the diagnostic criteria for standard PTSD (2021). Several studies have been done to test the validity of this distinction between PTSD and complex PTSD. These studies have found that the exposure to trauma and the symptoms of C-PTSD patients is different from standard PTSD. The patients that were diagnosed with complex PTSD had a longer exposure to trauma and more severe symptoms. Additionally, complex PTSD resulted in more functional impairment compared to PTSD (Ford and Courtois, 2021). The distinction of C-PTSD is important for those who live in a constant state of PTSD symptoms.

Even though the *ICD-11* recognizes complex PTSD as a different type of PTSD, the *DSM-V* does not. The *DSM-V* only describes PTSD as a single disorder. Within its diagnostic framework however, the *DSM-V* lists dissociative PTSD as a distinct subtype, which will be discussed later in the chapter. Moreover, the main way the *DSM-V* defines PTSD is under the singular term PTSD without additional types. In order to distinguish between different types of PTSD, the diagnostic criteria can be helpful in setting a basic framework of categorization. The *DSM-V* does not specifically outline types of PTSD, but rather has different criteria that must be met in order to receive a diagnosis. Each of the criteria list specific requirements or symptoms the patients must have in order to be diagnosed with PTSD (*DSM-V*, 2022). Moreover, these criteria can be used to establish differences within PTSD cases and further define any potential subtypes.

Foremost, an important criterion used to diagnose PTSD is criterion A. Criterion A refers to one of the eight criteria curated by the *DSM-V* in order to diagnose PTSD. In order to be diagnosed with PTSD, a patient should have at least one symptom from criterion A, which is the presence of a stressor (*DSM-V*, 2022). The main rationale behind PTSD is the exposure to a stressor that results in psychopathology. While the trauma and psychopathology experienced from the stressor or traumatic event can be common across PTSD cases, the stressor varies from case to case. While the differences in stressors are not considered subtypes of PTSD, there are several types of stressors that are commonly experienced by PTSD patients. The first distinction between stressors is the type of exposure. Exposure to a traumatic event or stressor can be of two types: direct exposure and indirect exposure. In terms of *direct exposure*, it can be defined as having direct exposure and involvement with the stressor. Some examples include being a victim of abuse, being involved in a life-threatening accident, etc. On the other side, indirect exposure is when an individual is not directly exposed to or involved with the stressor. Some examples of this can include learning of a traumatic experience that has occurred to a loved one, watching a traumatic event, etc. While the *DSM-5* does not make a distinction between the intensity and period of exposure, some studies have shown that exposure can have implications for PTSD prognosis. A review done on exposure and trauma found that there is a lower risk of developing PTSD from indirect exposure compared to direct exposure ("Direct vs. Indirect Exposure," 2021). Additionally, the type of exposure can also lead to different impact levels. Therefore, differences in exposure may lead to different prognosis for PTSD.

There are three groups of people known to experience the most complicated and extreme cases of PTSD: Adults who have gone through a rough childhood, who then experience another trauma as an adult, sexual assault survivors, and war veterans. Usually, these individuals not only have PTSD symptoms, but also are likely to develop other mental health issues such as thoughts of suicide, alcohol and substance abuse, depression, and other forms of anxiety.

CHILDHOOD TRAUMA SURVIVORS

Childhood trauma may consist of mental, physical, or sexual abuse, and extends to neglect and abandonment. Children that have had one of these experiences are more than likely to either develop PTSD from a very young age or go through PTSD in their adult life after experiencing any scale of trauma in their adult life. They are likely to go through more severe forms of PTSD. This can be due to partaking in behavior that can lead to more trauma after the experience in their childhood. For example, an individual may try to cope with their emotional trauma by taking drugs to numb the pain. In order to obtain the drugs, they place themselves in unfortunate and dangerous circumstances. These risky situations increase the likelihood of being abused, harmed directly, or watching indirectly. These experiences cause the individual to become further traumatized.

SEXUAL ASSAULT SURVIVORS

Sexual assault has been defined as any form of sexual activity that involves one or more people forcing another to engage in one or more sexual acts or behaviors against his or her own will. Rape has been as the most common form of sexual assault. Nonetheless, it is important to know that sexual assault is not limited to actual intercourse, such as the penetration of the vagina. Sexual assault can also be identified as verbal and emotional acts of assault. The mass media has led society to believe that only females can be victims of sexual assault—this is incorrect. Both men and women can be victims of sexual assault and can be affected by PTSD.

Many individuals have questioned how PTSD can be a result of sexual assault. It should be enough that their body has been harmed and taken advantage of, but it is also mentally damaging. Victims of sexual assault have been betrayed in very intimate and personal ways. It is generally believed by everyone that the people closest to them can be trusted. It is also common to have at least a basic level of trust out of courtesy to strangers. As children we are taught the golden rule: "Treat others as we expect to be treated." This statement hardly feels true after experiencing an assault. The victims' trust is challenged and changed.

Although both sexes can become victims of sexual assault, women are more likely to be the victims. The rest of this section will focus on how women are affected. To understand how women become victims of PTSD, it is important to try and comprehend what women go through prior to becoming a victim.

For many women that have experienced any form of sexual assault, it is likely that they have been assaulted by someone they know rather than a stranger. In adulthood, these women can become victims of assault again by people they have a relationship with, such as a husband, boyfriend, or a former intimate partner. Unfortunately, for many of these women, they tend to be attracted to abusive men.

For women who have experienced sexual assault, sex has the potential to lose its sensuality and feel rough, aggressive, or even terrifying. These women cannot usually identify "red flag" scenarios as easily because they have never been a part of a healthy relationship. This usually occurs because the women have been abused by people, they thought they could trust, people who were supposed to love them. As a result, women who have suffered sexual abuse, often do not realize what a good relationship should be.

Unfortunately, due to this lack of understanding of intimate sexual relationships, women who have suffered sexual assault can find it hard to say "no" to forms of sexual advances. In a relationship, these women become sexually objectified and are easily manipulated to perform sexual acts, even if they have little interest in the suggested activities. A detrimental aspect of this type of relationship is that women are led to believe that they were taking part in a consensual sexual encounter. Some women who were abused in their childhood even attempt to change the outcome of the abusive situation by recreating it. They purposefully place themselves in similar conditions and try to take control. But often these women fall prey to the same outcome. This outcome of course is only another form of stressor which can work to trigger PTSD.

Some women will take an opposite approach to the trauma of sexual assault and choose instead to isolate themselves. In order to fill the void created by lack of human contact, these individuals often turn to illicit chemical substances, alcohol, food, and even choose to take life-threatening risks. By turning to these situations, as an attempt to deal with their emotional problems, this places individuals in scenarios similar to their first sexual assault and the chances of reexperiencing some form of assault becomes greater.

WAR SURVIVORS

Furthermore, another aspect of the stressor involved in PTSD is that it can vary considerably from case to case with different implications. While the presence of any stressor that leads to trauma can be potentially psychopathological, some stressors can lead to varied or more severe symptoms ("Direct vs. Indirect Exposure," 2021). One category of stressors that have been seen to cause PTSD in war veterans are military and war related traumas. Despite the fact that war veterans are diagnosed and treated under most of the same frameworks as civilian populations, many studies have found that war veterans experience PTSD differently. One study found that war veterans experience PTSD at higher rates compared to the general population ("How Common Is PTSD in Adults?" n.d.). Additionally, another article exploring traumatic brain injury (TBI) found that TBI led to a higher risk of PTSD in military veterans compared to civilian populations (Loignon et al., 2020). Therefore, war veterans' PTSD is one of the major common categories of PTSD.

ABUSE SURVIVORS

In addition to this, another prevalent form of trauma or stressor is abuse. This abuse can be further form categories such as emotional abuse, psychological abuse, physical abuse, etc. Additionally, it can also branch out to domestic abuse, sexual abuse, childhood abuse. Each of these stressors has specific impacts on the type and severity of PTSD symptoms. For example, a study was done to explore the treatment and severity of symptoms of PTSD from parental emotional abuse. The study found that emotional abuse led to the most severe PTSD symptoms across different types of parental abuse (Hoeboer et al., 2021). Therefore, while

PTSD does not have trauma-based subtypes, there are still differences within how each trauma impacts the prognosis of PTSD.

Additionally, another distinction the *DSM-V* makes within PTSD cases is criterion B: Intrusion symptoms (*DSM-V*, 2022). In terms of symptomatology, each case of PTSD will have its own unique set of symptoms. This is mainly due to the variance that exists in the development and prognosis of psychopathology in the first place. Similar to the trauma section, the intrusive symptom section also contains variance in how each symptom is presented within each case. For example, some of the intrusion symptoms listed by the *DSM-V* include intrusive memories, nightmares, flashbacks, emotional or physical distress upon recalling the traumatic event, and so on (*DSM-V*, 2022). While these symptoms may exist differently across PTSD cases, it is possible for certain types of symptoms to exist within specific cases. Similarly, other criteria from the *DSM-V* also have subtypes and heterogeneity within them that can be employed to categorize different types of PTSD. Likewise, other criteria such as negative alterations in cognition and arousal also have differences in how they are presented across different cases. For example, some stressors may produce more severe alterations compared to others.

Furthermore, another subtype or specification the *DSM-V* makes is delayed-onset PTSD. The *DSM-V* states that any PTSD that is diagnosed after six months of the initial experience of trauma is classified under the delayed onset specification. In such cases, the patients do not show PTSD symptoms immediately after being exposed to a traumatic situation and symptoms usually appear much later (*DSM-V*, 2022). While the *DSM-V* considers this a specification, many studies have been done on the validity of this classification. In a study done on delayed onset, it was found that delayed onset may have been utilized and specified due to definition and diagnostic criteria confusions. Similarly, to further explore the subtype of delayed onset, another study on delayed onset stated that military veterans have more cases of delayed onset compared to civilian populations. The study highlighted that delayed PTSD could possibly happen from many different underlying neurobiological mechanisms (Smid et al., 2022). Therefore, the subtype of delayed onset of PTSD is highlighted in the *DSM-V* and can be used to distinguish it from standard PTSD. The acceptability of this type is low and is still a topic of exploration.

In addition to the aforementioned classifications, one of the distinctions that the *DSM-V* makes within its classification of posttraumatic stress disorder symptoms is the symptom of dissociation (*DSM-V,* 2022). The dissociation subtype of PTSD is mainly characterized by depersonalization and derealization in addition to the standard PTSD diagnostic criteria.

Depersonalization can be defined as a feeling of detachment and dissociation from oneself and environment. Similarly, derealization can be defined as the feeling that reality does not exist or is unreal. Dissociative PTSD has been seen to be distinct from PTSD for additional reasons as well.

Similarly, another potential subtype of PTSD is comorbid PTSD. While PTSD is a single disorder on its own, often it exists with other comorbid psychopathologies. Studies have shown that almost 80% of adults with PTSD have mentioned, at minimum, one other comorbid disorder (Fox et al., 2020). There is also a higher instance of comorbidity noticed in those who suffered spousal abuse (Fox et al., 2020). The reason why it is necessary to distinguish comorbid PTSD from a single PTSD diagnosis is to be able to better determine the prognosis, or potential treatment outcome of the patient. In terms of PTSD, one of the most prevalent forms of comorbidity occurs with major depressive disorder, with 30%-50% of the people with PTSD also being diagnosed with major depressive disorder (Angelakis et al., 2020). Additionally, other forms of comorbidity may have developed as a result of trying to cope with the patient's trauma. For example, several studies have tried to explore whether substance abuse comorbidity is a result of trying to cope with trauma in PTSD patients. Similarly, in childhood abuse cases almost all children end up developing a comorbid condition. Therefore, it is essential to distinguish comorbid PTSD from singular PTSD so questions and concerns like these can be considered when developing treatments and directing research on PTSD.

While the aforementioned terms describe anomalies and complex cases of PTSD, another interesting way to define PTSD is the use of the term uncomplicated PTSD. While there is no official definition of uncomplicated PTSD, it is used to describe a low intensity type of PTSD. It is employed to highlight cases of PTSD that may not have as severe symptoms as other cases ("Types of PTSD," n.d.). While this grouping also includes PTSD symptoms and treatment methods, the prognosis is seen to be short lived with very high rates of treatment success. This, however, is not a formal term employed by clinicians. Building upon the theme of severity and intensity of prognosis, another proposed subtype of PTSD is based upon personalities. Researchers have formulated three different subtypes of PTSD that are based on the personality of the patient. The three subtypes are known as internalizing PTSD, externalizing PTSD, and low pathology PTSD (Egerton et al., 2019). Furthermore, internalizers are generally individuals with PTSD with higher experiences of negative emotions including but not limited to anxiety, depression, and more. (Panuccio et al., 2022). In contrast to internalizers, externalizers were more aggressive. They are more likely to behave aggressively, delinquently, and have issues with authority and social conduct. It was also found that the higher the quantity of traumas, the more likely young adult patients would develop externalized symptoms of PTSD (Panuccio et al., 2022). Lastly, some other ways to differentiate between different types of PTSD presentations is distinguishing based on biological and social characteristics such as sex, age, ethnicity, and genetics. Similarly, several studies have found that females are at a higher risk of developing PTSD more than men. For example, one such study estimated that women were two or three times more likely to be diagnosed with PTSD than men (Vogt, n.d.). Additionally, there has also been research on ethnicity that may impact the prognosis and experience of a PTSD patient. Several studies have focused on ethnicity and found that sometimes ethnicity may increase the risk of developing PTSD. A combination of social and cultural differences, as well as specific ethnic differences proves significant in the disparities of PTSD in different cultures (Spoont and McClendon, 2020). Overall, these studies and observations conclude that PTSD can have additional subgroups and categories.

As discussed throughout this chapter, there are not specified types of PTSD which can make it difficult to categorize it further. The main reason behind the lack of subtypes within PTSD is the heterogeneity and diversity in its onset and prognosis. The experience of trauma and finding something traumatic can be a very personalized experience which can be difficult to capture through one specific standardized method. Even with a large amount of knowledge and research on the topic of PTSD, its diagnostic criteria and categorizations are constantly being updated as more discoveries and advancements are made. Therefore, at present while the *DSM* and *ICD-11* only add or specify a few sub-types of PTSD, there are still prevalent themes across certain traumas and symptoms that can be further classified into types. Not only will this make classification easier but will also aid in more specification in research and treatments. In essence, PTSD is presented in many different ways and can have several different subtypes. In addition, PTSD is still a fairly new psychopathology and is still being explored.

REFERENCES

Angelakis, S., N. Weber, and R. D. V. Nixon. "Comorbid Posttraumatic Stress Disorder and Major Depressive Disorder: The Usefulness of a Sequential Treatment Approach within a Randomised Design." *Journal of Anxiety Disorders* 76: 102324, December 2020. https://doi.org/10.1016/j.janxdis.2020.102324

Bovin, M. J., A. A. Camden, and F. W. Weathers. "Literature on DSM-5 and ICD-11: An Update." *PTSD Research Quarterly* 32, no. 2, 2021

Cloitre, M. "ICD-11 Complex Post-Traumatic Stress Disorder: Simplifying Diagnosis in Trauma Populations." *The British Journal of Psychiatry* 216, no. 3: 129–31, 2020. https://doi.org/10.1192/bjp.2020.43

Diagnostic and Statistical Manual of Mental Disorders: DSM-5-TR (DSM-V). American Psychiatric Association Publishing, 2022.

"Direct vs. Indirect Exposure." NeuRA Library, October 8, 2021. https://library.neura.edu.au/ptsd-library/risk-factors-ptsd-library/trauma-characteristics/direct-vs-indirect-exposure/index.html#:~:text=Moderate%20quality%20evidence%20finds%20the,friends%20%3D%203%2D13.8%25)

Egerton, G. A., S. A. Radomski, and J. P. Read. "Personality-Based Posttraumatic Stress Disorder Subtypes in Young Adults." *Traumatology* 25, no. 4: 235–41, December 2019. https://doi.org/10.1037/trm0000185

Ford, J. D., and C. A. Courtois. "Complex PTSD and Borderline Personality Disorder." *Borderline Personality Disorder and Emotion Dysregulation* 8, no. 1, May 6, 2021. https://doi.org/10.1186/s40479-021-00155-9

Fox, R., P. Hyland, J. M. Power, and A. N. Coogan. "Patterns of Comorbidity Associated with ICD-11 PTSD among Older Adults in the United States." *Psychiatry Research* 290: 113171, August 2020. https://doi.org/10.1016/j.psychres.2020.113171

Hoeboer, C., C. de Roos, G. van Son, P. Spinhoven, and B. Elzinga. "The Effect of Parental Emotional Abuse on the Severity and Treatment of PTSD Symptoms in Children and Adolsecents." *Child Abuse & Neglect* 111: 104775, January 2021. https://doi.org/10.1016/j.chiabu.2020.104775

"How Common Is PTSD in Adults?" U.S. Department of Veterans Affairs, n.d. https://www.ptsd.va.gov/understand/common/common_adults.asp#:~:text=About%205%20out%20of%20every,some%20point%20in%20their%20life

ICD-11. *ICD-11 for Mortality and Morbidity Statistics*. World Health Organization, 2019. https://icd.who.int/browse11/l-m/en#/http://id.who.int/icd/entity/585833559

Loignon, A., M. Ouellet, and G. Belleville. "A Systematic Review and Meta-analysis on PTSD Following TBI Among Military/Veteran and Civilian Populations." *Journal of Head Trauma Rehabilitation* m35, no. 1, E21–E35, 2020. https://doi.org/10.1097/htr.0000000000000514

Mayo Clinic Staff. "Post-Traumatic Stress Disorder (PTSD)." Mayo Clinic, December 13, 2022. https://www.mayoclinic.org/diseases-conditions/post-traumatic-stress-disorder/symptoms-causes/syc-20355967#:~:text=Post%2Dtraumatic%20stress%20disorder%20(PTSD)%20is%20a%20mental%20health,uncontrollable%20thoughts%20about%20the%20event

"Neurobiology of Trauma." University of Northern Colorado, n.d. https://www.unco.edu/assault-survivors-advocacy-program/learn_more/neurobiology_of_trauma.aspxPanuccio, A., D. Biondo, E. Picerni, B. Genovesi, and D. Laricchiuta. "Trauma-Related Internalizing and Externalizing Behaviors in Adolescence: A Bridge between Psychoanalysis and Neuroscience." *Adolescents* 2, no. 4: 413–23, September 21, 2022. https://doi.org/10.3390/adolescents2040032

Smid, G. E., J. Lind, and J. P. Bonde. "Neurobiological Mechanisms Underlying Delayed Expression of Posttraumatic Stress Disorder: A Scoping Review." *World Journal of Psychiatry* 12, no. 1: 151–68, January 19, 2022. https://doi.org/10.5498/wjp.v12.i1.151

Spoont, M., and J. McClendon. "Racial and Ethnic Disparities in PTSD." *PTSD Research Quarterly* 31, no. 4, 2020. https://www.ptsd.va.gov/publications/rq_docs/V31N4.pdf

"Types of PTSD." Black Bear Lodge, n.d. https://blackbearrehab.com/mental-health/ptsd/types-of-ptsd/

Vogt, D. "Research on Women, Trauma and PTSD." U.S. Department of Veterans Affairs, n.d. https://www.ptsd.va.gov/professional/treat/specific/ptsd_research_women.asp#:~:text=Estimates%20from%20community%20studies%20suggest,%25%20for%20men%20(5)

CHAPTER 8

THE PHYSIOLOGICAL, PSYCHOLOGICAL, AND BEHAVIORAL RESPONSE TO TRAUMA AND PTSD

Posttraumatic stress disorder (PTSD) is a mental health condition caused by a traumatic or life-altering event (Mann and Marwaha, 2023). Such events can include experiencing a natural disaster, extreme violence or being abused. The effects of PTSD can implicate a person on a physiological, psychological, and behavior level (Mann and Marwaha, 2023). Physiological effects often start as experiencing a racing heart rate, fatigue, and progress to contributing to long-term physical severe conditions such as coronary artery disease, hypertension, and hyperlipidemia. Also, advanced research is exploring the exact mechanisms and means by which PTSD can go about the increased risk for disease and causing permanent physiological changes. Furthermore, PTSD is often primarily defined in psychology, and therefore, someone with PTSD experiences a variety of psychological symptoms. Symptoms often correlate with the stages of trauma, with a critical hallmark of PTSD symptomology being flashbacks. Lastly, considering the immense effects PTSD has on the body and mind, it also has a significant impact on the behaviors of an individual. PTSD can severely hinder an individual's ability to maintain productivity, personality, and health. Ultimately, PTSD is circular in that many implications of PTSD impact an individual's family. Overall, PTSD is a serious condition that intimately impacts an individual in physical, psychological, and behavioral ways and operates in a vicious cycle that proceeds to impact family members and perhaps transgress to future generations. Therefore, PTSD needs to be prioritized in order to ensure a mentally and physically healthier tomorrow.

To begin with, many mental conditions such as PTSD have physiological implications. Such implications can begin in the form of an increased heart rate, feelings of fatigue, muscle tension, aches and pains, and insomnia (Mann and Marwaha, 2023). Although, in most extreme and long-term cases, research has proposed correlations between PTSD patients and increased chance of more serious physical conditions such as hypertension, hyperlipidemia, and coronary artery disease. These physiological effects can severely impact an individual's ability to operate in society and can proceed to negatively impact one's behavior and psychological state. Also, physiological changes can occur to the brain and genome as a repercussion of PTSD (Mann and Marwaha, 2023). Therefore, although the scope of physical implications to PTSD is enormous, all symptoms should be treated with the utmost care as patients with minor physical symptoms can still progress to extreme and irreversible consequences.

For instance, one study recruited 141 current and former U.S. service members from a military treatment facility to investigate posttraumatic stress disorder (PTSD) and its relationship with sleep quality (Biggs et al., 2020). Participants completed a questionnaire-based assessment to determine exposure to traumatic events, with all participants reporting at least one qualifying traumatic exposure. The severity of PTSD symptoms was evaluated using the 20-item PCL-5 questionnaire. Participants rated each item based on symptom severity, with responses ranging from 0 (Not at all) to 4 (Extremely). A diagnosis of probable PTSD was made according to *DSM-V* criteria, requiring specific symptom clusters and a minimum symptom severity score of 38. Regarding sleep assessment, participants reported their sleep duration, number of awakenings during the night, and overall sleep quality. Sleep duration and number of awakenings were measured through surveys. Sleep quality was evaluated using a single item adapted from the

Pittsburgh Sleep Quality Index (PSQI), where participants rated their overall sleep quality on a scale ranging from 0 (Very bad) to 3 (Very good). Furthermore, sleep problems such as trouble falling asleep and difficulty staying asleep were assessed using a set of 20 items adapted from various sources, including the PCL-5 and PSQI, or developed specifically for this study. Participants indicated whether they experienced each sleep problem the previous night, with response options of 0 (No) or 1 (Yes). Overall, the study's findings suggest that sleep disturbances, including sleep duration, trouble falling asleep, and difficulty staying asleep, vary from night to night and are associated with subsequent changes in PTSD symptoms. The assessment tools utilized provided insight into both the severity of PTSD symptoms and various aspects of sleep quality, highlighting the complex interplay between sleep and PTSD (Biggs et al., 2020).

Furthermore, in a retrospective longitudinal cohort study involving U.S. women veterans enrolled in Veterans Health Administration care, Ebrahimi et al. (2024) investigated the association between PTSD and incident ischemic heart disease (IHD). Utilizing electronic health records (I), propensity score matching was employed to pair women with PTSD to those without PTSD based on various factors. Cox regression analysis was then utilized to explore the time until the diagnosis of incident IHD, including coronary artery disease, angina, or myocardial infarction, with PTSD and potential mediating risk factors considered (Ebrahimi et al., 2024). The study, building on prior research indicating a 44% greater rate of incident IHD among women veterans with PTSD, delved into specific mechanisms linking PTSD to IHD and their relative contributions. Notably, PTSD was associated with increased rates of various risk factors, with psychiatric disorders playing a significant role in mediating the association between PTSD and IHD. Specifically, psychiatric disorders accounted for a larger proportion of the PTSD-IHD link compared to traditional risk factors. The findings underscore the importance of addressing both PTSD and its psychiatric comorbidities when evaluating cardiovascular risk in patients with PTSD, given their high prevalence (Ebrahimi et al., 2024). Understanding the underlying mechanisms and exploring potential interventions, including psychotherapies, pharmacotherapies, and transdiagnostic treatments, is crucial for mitigating cardiovascular risk in this population.

In a separate study, subjects were recruited from a postdeployment mental health repository of 3877 US military Veterans between 2005 and 2018. The study focused on Veterans aged 18 to 59 who served since September 11, 2001, and underwent screening for inclusion and exclusion criteria, including PTSD and comorbid major depression (Clausen et al., 2020). A total of 341 Veterans met the inclusion criteria for analysis, all of whom provided written informed consent. The study aimed to investigate the impact of combat exposure on neural health in a sample of combat Veterans (N = 337). Results revealed that combat exposure severity, independent of PTSD, was associated with lower cortical thickness in various regions of the left prefrontal lobe, including the rostral middle frontal, superior frontal, medial orbitofrontal, and rostral anterior cingulate cortices. Additionally, combat exposure severity was linked to increased cortical thickness in the left middle and inferior temporal cortex. Notably, PTSD was associated with lower cortical thickness in the right fusiform extending into the lateral occipital and inferior temporal cortex. This suggests that PTSD has a distinct impact on cortical thickness in specific brain regions among combat Veterans (Clausen et al., 2020). Furthermore, Veterans who sustained head injuries exhibited increased cortical thickness bilaterally in the medial prefrontal cortex, indicating a separate effect of head injuries on cortical thickness (Clausen et al., 2020). These findings highlight the complex interplay between combat exposure severity, PTSD, and head injuries in influencing cortical thickness in Veteran populations.

Significant atrophy of the brain is a physiological symptom of PTSD, but because structure dictates function, losing significant brain volume can lead to many psychological and behavioral effects. An example of an effect could be the loss of cognitive flexibility, as demonstrated by a study investigating cognitive decline in Veterans with PTSD (Prieto et al., 2023). Subjects for this study were recruited from a postdeployment mental health repository of US Vietnam War Veterans between 2005 and 2018. The study aimed to investigate the association between PTSD symptoms, Alzheimer's disease (AD) biomarkers, and cognitive function over time (Prieto et al., 2023). Three main findings emerged from the analysis of 337 Veterans: first, PTSD symptom severity was associated with cognitive decline on both the MMSE and the MoCA, especially in the attention and memory domains. Second, PTSD symptom severity significantly predicted decline in cognition, even after accounting for factors such as age, education, and history of traumatic brain injury (TBI). Third, no relationships were found between AD biomarkers and change in cognitive function. These results support previous findings indicating a link between PTSD symptom severity and cognitive decline, emphasizing the importance of considering traumatic stress when examining cognitive function. Although the effect size is relatively small, likely due to the short follow-up period, the findings highlight the potential impact of PTSD symptoms on cognitive health in aging Veterans (Prieto et al., 2023). Several explanations have been proposed for the association between PTSD and cognitive symptoms, including stress-induced glucocorticoid dysregulation, reduced cognitive and brain reserve, and sleep impairments. Anatomical differences in PTSD, such as smaller hippocampal volume and cortical thinning in the medial prefrontal cortex, may also contribute to cognitive decline (Prieto et al., 2023). Thus, considering PTSD symptoms in cognitive assessments may improve the identification and management of cognitive decline in aging Veterans with a history of trauma.

In addition, although the immense example of loss of cognitive flexibility can be a cost of PTSD, some more mild symptoms that often coincide with the initial stages following a traumatic event include shock, denial, anxiety, guilt, fear, blame, irritability, and confusion (Mann and Marwaha, 2023). These emotions, if ignored, can continue to burden an individual and impact their day-to-day life and productivity. Also, one of the most common psychological symptoms of PTSD is having flashbacks of the past traumatic event. Flashbacks can be very uncomfortable and frightening for an individual with PTSD as it puts them back in that space of abuse or violence. Eventually, one can develop more severe psychological or mental health-related conditions such as depression which can seriously escalate the mental toll PTSD can have on a person. Overall, the psychological impact of PTSD is tied to the physical and biological changes due to PTSD.

Moreover, PTSD can have many behavioral implications intimately associated with the physiological and psychological burden they place on an individual. Such implications can include lack of productivity and attendance in work and school, the development of self-destructive tendencies, and aggressive behavior (Mann and Marwaha, 2023). Specifically, PTSD has immense consequences for the body and mind, and these implications can seriously hinder one's ability to be productive and go to school or work. Also, PTSD can drive people into addictions as an attempt to cope with their past trauma. PTSD can also drive people to be more aggressive, and perhaps this could put their colleagues and family members at risk of being abused. The idea of being abusive as a response to trauma also contributes to the circular nature of PTSD. Lastly, PTSD can prompt one to return to past events or relive past trauma in the form of seeking similar relationships and opportunities to be a victim. Overall, there are many behavioral implications for an individual suffering from PTSD and this can result in family members not even recognizing their loved one due to their significant changes in personality and temperament.

A significant implication of PTSD on the behavior of an individual is frequently their ability to be productive. A specific study attempting to examine the relationship between PTSD symptomology and return to usual major activity for postsecondary students should be considered when evaluating the loss of productivity due to PTSD (Vilaplana-Pérez et al., 2020). The study examined the educational outcomes of individuals in Sweden born between 1973 and 1997, totaling 2,551,071 individuals. Exclusions were made for various factors, resulting in a final cohort of 2,244,193 individuals followed until 2013 for their educational attainment. Individuals diagnosed with PTSD were significantly less likely to achieve educational milestones compared to those without PTSD. For instance, those diagnosed with PTSD before completing compulsory education had significantly lower odds of accessing upper secondary education. Similarly, individuals diagnosed with PTSD during different age intervals had markedly lower odds of completing upper secondary education or starting/finishing a university degree compared to their peers without PTSD. Notably, there were no observed sex differences in these educational outcomes. Even after adjusting for factors such as familial influences, psychiatric comorbidity, and cognitive ability, the association between PTSD and impaired educational performance persisted (Vilaplana-Pérez et al., 2020). This underscores the need for trauma-informed interventions in educational settings to mitigate the long-term socioeconomic impact of academic underachievement.

For example, a study examined 189 young adults, predominantly with current PTSD and AUD, who had experienced interpersonal trauma and engaged in weekly alcohol use. Participants underwent a trauma and alcohol cue reactivity assessment, measuring subjective and physiological responses to personalized trauma and alcohol cues (Berenz et al., 2021). Results from linear mixed-effects models revealed that trauma cue-elicited craving was higher among individuals with elevated PTSD symptoms, a finding consistent with previous research. Notably, this elevated craving was fully accounted for by increases in negative affect, with no direct effect of trauma cues on craving observed (Berenz et al., 2021). Furthermore, PTSD symptoms moderated the association between trauma cues and negative affect, while coping motives for alcohol moderated the association between negative affect and craving. These findings highlight the significant role of negative affect, PTSD symptoms, and coping motives in alcohol craving among trauma-exposed individuals with AUD. The study provides valuable insights for understanding the mechanisms underlying alcohol craving in this population and suggests avenues for developing interventions targeting negative reinforcement drinking in those with comorbid PTSD and AUD. Overall, the study emphasizes that a relationship between PTSD and alcohol exists, and this relationship should be further explored as well as the general relationship between PTSD and addictive behaviors.

Additionally, the behavioral impact of PTSD can also impact the loved ones of the affected. For instance, a study by Schwartz et al. (2021) focused on the experiences of 36 family members of Canadian Armed Forces (CAF) Veterans living with mental health issues. These family members, including spouses, siblings, parents, and adult children, were recruited through various channels, such as Military Family Resource Centres, Operational Stress Injury Support Services clinics, and social media. The findings revealed that navigating the Military Casualty Treatment (MCT) process alongside a Veteran with significant mental health issues was challenging for family members (Schwartz et al., 2021). They encountered barriers such as stigma, confidentiality concerns, exclusion from administrative processes, and lack of awareness, leading to increased feelings of isolation and helplessness. Family members described their experiences as disorienting and burdensome, especially as they struggled to access informal and formal resources critical for adjusting to civilian life. Many were providing essential care for daily activities, exacerbating caregiver burden. While family and friends were primary sources of informal support, stigma and privacy concerns sometimes hindered their ability to provide effective care. Thus, this study demonstrates the immense cost of PTSD for those involved and ultimately makes PTSD become more of a family issue rather than the issue of a single individual (Schwartz et al., 2021).

In conclusion, there is an intimate connection between PTSD and physiological, psychological, and behavioral implications. Specifically, PTSD can manifest in many physiological symptoms such as fatigue, an increase in heart rate, and insomnia (Mann and Marwaha, 2023). The physiological repercussions however can become increasingly more severe in the long term and include an increased risk of heart disease, for instance (Ebrahimi et al., 2024). Additionally, as research continues, links will continue to be established between PTSD and gray matter brain atrophy and mechanisms by which PTSD wreaks havoc on the body and mind, such as biomarkers. Similar to the physiological symptoms of PTSD, there are several quintessentially telling psychological symptoms such as shock, denial, fear, anxiety, and irritability (Mann and Marwaha, 2023). In the long term, however, PTSD can be the root of mental illness. Due to the immense role of an individual physically and mentally, it is logical also to see an individual affected by PTSD behaving differently. Such behaviors can include a lack of productivity, the adoption of self-destructive habits, aggressive behaviors, and the constant need to repeat past experiences of trauma. Ironically, the behaviors caused by PTSD can easily perpetuate the cycle of damage for an individual, their loved ones, and potentially future generations (Schwartz et al., 2021). Overall, PTSD is a severe condition that can destroy an individual physically and mentally and cause them to behave in a way that compromises their productivity, personality, and future. That is why people need to be aware of this pressing issue and act today to help themselves and others maintain good health.

REFERENCES

Berenz, E. C., S. Edalatian Zakeri, A. P. Demos, K. C. Paltell, H. Bing-Canar, S. Kevorkian, and R. Ranney. "Negative Affect and Alcohol Craving in Trauma-Exposed Young Adult Drinkers." *Alcoholism: Clinical and Experimental Research*, 45(7), 1479–1493, 2021. https://doi.org/10.1111/acer.14641.

Biggs, Q. M., R. J. Ursano, J. Wang, G. H. Wynn, R. B. Carr, and C. S. Fullerton. "Post Traumatic Stress Symptom Variation Associated with Sleep Characteristics." BMC Psychiatry, 20(1), 2020. https://doi.org/10.1186/s12888-020-02550-y.

Clausen, A. N., E. Clarke, R. D. Phillips, C. Haswell, and R. A. Morey. "Combat Exposure, Posttraumatic Stress Disorder, and Head Injuries Differentially Relate to Alterations in Cortical Thickness in Military Veterans." Neuropsychopharmacology, 45(3), 491–498, 2020. https://doi.org/10.1038/s41386-019-0539-9.

Ebrahimi, R., P. A. Dennis, A. Laurie, C. H. Tseng, C. A. Alvarez, J. C. Beckham, and J. A. Sumner. "Pathways Linking Posttraumatic Stress Disorder to Incident Ischemic Heart Disease in Women." JACC, 3(1), 100744–100744, 2024. https://doi.org/10.1016/j.jacadv.2023.100744.

Mann, S. K., and R. Marwaha. "Posttraumatic Stress Disorder (PTSD)." PubMed; StatPearls Publishing, January 30, 2023. https://www.ncbi.nlm.nih.gov/books/NBK559129/.

Prieto, S., K. E. Nolan, J. N. Moody, S. M. Hayes, and J. P. Hayes. "Posttraumatic Stress Symptom Severity Predicts Cognitive Decline Beyond the Effect of Alzheimer's Disease Biomarkers in Veterans." Translational Psychiatry, 13(1), 1–9, 2023. https://doi.org/10.1038/s41398-023-02354-0.

Schwartz, K. D., D. Norris, H. Cramm, L. Tam-Seto, and A. Mahar. "Family Members of Veterans with Mental Health Problems: Seeking, Finding, and Accessing Informal and Formal Supports During the Military-to-Civilian Transition." *Journal of Military, Veteran and Family Health*. e20190023, 2021. https://doi.org/10.3138/jmvfh-2019-0023.

Vilaplana-Pérez, A., A. Sidorchuk, A. Pérez-Vigil, G. Brander, K. Isoumura, E. Hesselmark, L. Sevilla-Cermeño, U. A. Valdimarsdóttir, H. Song, A. Jangmo, R. Kuja-Halkola, B. M. D'Onofrio, H. Larsson, G. Garcia-Soriano, D. Mataix-Cols, and L. Fernández de la Cruz. "Assessment of Posttraumatic Stress Disorder and Educational Achievement in Sweden." JAMA Network Open, 3(12), e2028477, 2020. https://doi.org/10.1001/jamanetworkopen.2020.28477.

CHAPTER 9

SYMPTOMS OF *PTSD*

Psychiatrists have stated that PTSD should only be diagnosed after several months have elapsed after the trauma has occurred (Bhandari, 2022). Without a formal diagnosis being established by a psychiatrist, the individual is deemed to be experiencing post-traumatic stress related to the event. To be formally diagnosed, the patient must display symptoms from three categories that differentiate PTSD from other mental health problems (Mann and Marwaha, 2023). The first category of symptoms involves the victim reexperiencing the traumatic event, often at nighttime. The second category is based on reclusive behavior, PTSD victims avoid social and public interaction, when possible, to prevent the possibility of being in contact with stimuli related to their trauma. Stimuli may include sights, sounds, smells, or textures. In addition to antisocial behavior, sufferers are also likely to show a lack of interest in their surroundings. The third category is hyperarousal. Hyperarousal causes victims to be more irritable and to have interruptions in their sleep patterns. The individual is often unable to stay asleep or even fall asleep. This symptom is usually experienced immediately after the trauma, but it is also possible to experience it sometime after as a delayed onset of PTSD.

REEXPERIENCING SYMPTOMS

"Reexperiencing symptoms" is one of the most commonly depicted symptoms of PTSD and most of the public is aware of this aspect of the disorder. They are *flashbacks* and are the most problematic symptom of PTSD for sufferers, in particular for war veterans. *Reexperiencing* consists of recurring nightmares and experiencing strong distress. Physiologically, distress causes an increased heart rate, profuse sweating. During the flashbacks, the sufferer relives the trauma as if it were happening, it is not a recollection of the event. These flashbacks can be unconsciously triggered. The individual may not be aware of what the stimuli is, but their mind subconsciously remembers. Most flashback scenarios are rare and typically brief. During the occurrences, many victims hear the sounds from the event, or images of dead bodies or situations; this is called hallucinatory phenomena.

AVOIDANCE SYMPTOMS

For many individuals suffering from PTSD, a major part of their lives becomes focused on avoiding anything that will remind them of the traumatic event. Many PTSD victims of sexual abuse avoid their immediate family members, such as parents or siblings. Combat war veterans with PTSD avoid the media because of the possible involvement of war or physical violence in its subject matter. This includes television programs, news, or movies. There are several different forms of avoidance that PTSD victims will undertake to shield themselves from the trauma stimuli. Subtle forms of avoidance tend to be used to prevent the people around them from being aware of the trauma they experienced. Avoiding eye contact with others is one of the ways. The victims' methods of avoidance, however, can be as obvious as not participating in any activities they feel would stimulate their physiological experience during the trauma. Young children that have been sexually abused have the experience of an attacker forcing their body into hyperarousal. After the trauma, the abused children avoid physical activities that encourage a change in their physiological state. War veterans with PTSD also try to refrain from physical activity that results in hyperarousal, shortness of breath, sweating, and dizziness.

HYPERAROUSAL

Hyperarousal causes the PTSD sufferer a lack of sleep. This includes initial insomnia; difficulty falling asleep, and middle insomnia; staying asleep at night. Initial insomnia is caused by the fear of terrifying nightmares in which they relive the trauma. According to some researchers, middle insomnia is a by-product of hyperarousal. Other researchers believe that middle insomnia is caused by recurring nightmares (Moawad, 2020).

Hyperarousal also causes hypervigilance; the PTSD victim is very cautious. They appear to be extremely alert. Hypervigilance is most conspicuous in public settings. An example of this could be where the individual chooses to sit in a restaurant. They will likely choose a table that has a good view of everyone in the restaurant and sit with their backs to the wall facing the door. At home, the individual will constantly check whether the windows and doors are secure and locked. This is most common for PTSD victims of sexual abuse or violence.

Hyperarousal also comes with a lack of concentration; more effort is needed to focus. It may be reading a book or watching a television program, but it is also difficult to follow along in a conversation. Issues with concentration are caused by trauma-related thoughts. Hypervigilance is also a factor related to the lack of focus because the PTSD individual is constantly cautious of their surroundings rather than the matter at hand. Insomnia also plays into this, being unable to sleep at night causes fatigue and tiredness during the daytime.

STARTLE RESPONSE

Startle response is mostly experienced by PTSD sufferers with road traffic trauma. This response is reported by individuals as feeling extremely "jumpy." After an episode, it takes a long time for their body to calm down. It is also difficult for the victim to drive in traffic after the trauma. Driving involves fast movement around them and triggers the startle response. PTSD-diagnosed drivers may slam on the brakes and lose control of the car easily.

REFERENCES

Bhandari, S., Ed. "Posttraumatic Stress Disorder (PTSD): Symptoms, Diagnosis, Treatment." WebMD, August 31, 2022. https://www.webmd.com/mental-health/post-traumatic-stress-disorder

Mann, S. K., and R. Marwaha. "Posttraumatic Stress Disorder." StatPearls [Internet], January 30, 2023. https://www.ncbi.nlm.nih.gov/books/NBK559129/

Moawad, H. "Insomnia Triggered by Nightmares: Evaluation and Treatment Options." *Psychiatric Times*, November 16, 2020. https://www.psychiatrictimes.com/view/insomnia-triggered-nightmares-evaluation-and-treatment-options

10

PTSD in Different Age Groups

As previously discussed, posttraumatic stress disorder (PTSD) is a psychiatric disorder that may develop after a person is exposed to exceptionally threatening or horrifying events. PTSD can be caused by a single traumatic event or by prolonged exposure to trauma, such as sexual abuse or violence in childhood. Many people, unfortunately, go through traumatic events in their life and hence they can develop PTSD. PTSD is not limited to any age and can affect anyone of any age. Additionally, predicting who will develop PTSD is a huge challenge since there is no way for a person to find out what and when they will go through a traumatic event in their life (Li et al., 2023). It is known through research that patients of all ages who are diagnosed with PTSD are at an increased risk of experiencing poor health, including somatoform, cardiorespiratory, musculoskeletal, gastrointestinal, and immunological disorders. Moreover, PTSD is strongly associated with substantial psychiatric comorbidity, increased risk of suicide, and economic hardships (Li et al., 2023). PTSD is very common and can stay with a person for the entirety of their life because one trigger can cause them to be reminded about their traumatic experience. In such instances, the recollection is vivid and leads to excruciating pain. The person with PTSD along with the support of their physician and therapist needs resilience to counteract symptoms.

In addition to the harms that PTSD causes, it also has a high incidence rate. According to Zai et al. (2022), PTSD has become a global health issue, and although prevalence rates vary, studies indicate it costs approximately \$521–\$19,435 USD per person annually. Furthermore, because of a lack of data on PTSD in Canada, the first genome-wide association study was conducted which explained PTSD related comorbid conditions. A sample of 19,669 Canadians were genotyped and used in single-marker analyzes to determine phenotypes for PTSD status. These results were compiled and resulted in finding that polygenic risk scores for major depressive disorder, schizophrenia, educational attainment, and insomnia were associated with all four measured PTSD genetic markers. It is important to note that only insomnia and educational attainment were statistically significant. Although this research is telling, to understand the role and extent of trauma and its correlates requires further research regarding polygenic risk scores (Zai et al., 2022). Yet, even without genetic predispositions, people can still be impacted by other comorbidities (Brouzos et al., 2022).

PTSD is not a condition that discriminates against age, sex, ethnicity, profession, race, socioeconomic background, or belief systems. It can affect anyone, and the core of PTSD is trauma. Trauma can be experienced by anyone through abuse, violence, sexual abuse, death of a loved one, bullying, natural disaster, threat, or injury. Most commonly, PTSD is associated with extremely severe events such as famine, mass shootings, or wars, but the condition can affect people and children with seemingly minor traumas and can be debilitating (Zaragoza Scherman et al., 2020). Many studies have been done to explore the association between PTSD and age. Additionally, they have also explored whether certain ages are more likely to develop PTSD compared to others. The results of these studies indicated that PTSD does not adhere to a single age limit for diagnosis. Moreover, unlike any other mental illness or neurodegenerative disorders, mood disorders, and personality disorders, PTSD is a cocktail of largely external factors and a small handful of internal factors, hence diagnosis is strictly based upon chance than it is in genetic susceptibility (Zaragoza Scherman et al., 2020). Additionally, PTSD is strongly associated and observed in populations living in dangerous or war-torn regions which causes an increased risk of developing PTSD than any age-related criteria. Nevertheless, experiencing traumatic events during childhood puts children at an extremely increased risk of developing PTSD as well as other mood and personality disorders compared to any other age group or adults (Zaragoza Scherman et al., 2020). Hence, this chapter shows PTSD occurrence in different age groups, how PTSD affects different age groups, PTSD similarities in each age group, and if treatment is the same for each age group. The age groups are children and young adolescents, adults, and the elderly.

Children and young adolescents are categorized in the 0–18 age group and this age group is vulnerable to PTSD as well as traumatic events since children are generally innocent and are thought to be easy targets. Unfortunately, in Canada, there are no official statistics available for PTSD in children and teens. The United States of America data, however, reports that at least 5% of children (one in twenty) aged between 13 and 18 suffer from PTSD symptoms and meet many of the conditions needed for a PTSD diagnosis (Brooks and Greenberg, 2024). In children, PTSD is more common in females than in males (Stanford Children's Health, n.d.). Children and young teens may experience stressful events that can greatly impact their behavior, feelings, and thoughts and most of the time children are able to recover (Centers for Disease Control and Prevention, 2021). If children experience severe stress, for example in the form of an injury, or from violence, sexual abuse, or death or threatened death of a family member or friend, they will be affected long term and are at a high risk of developing PTSD (Centers for Disease Control and Prevention, 2021).

Children who are diagnosed with PTSD experience symptoms such as reliving the event repeatedly in thought or play, nightmares and sleep issues, being upset when something triggers them to remember memories of the event, no positive emotions, sad and unhappy, angry and easily irritated, constantly looking for threats and easily being startled and scared, feeling helpless and hopeless, denying that the event happened, feeling numb, avoid talking to people associated with the event, and avoid places and things associated with the event (Centers for Disease Control and Prevention, 2021). If children show these symptoms for at least one month after the event, they are at a risk of being diagnosed with PTSD (Centers for Disease Control and Prevention, 2021). The most common events seen in children that lead them to develop PTSD are associated with physical, sexual, or emotional abuse. Some examples include being a victim of violence or witnessing violent crimes, death, or serious illness of a close loved one such as a family member or a friend, manmade or natural disasters, and car accidents (Centers for Disease Control and Prevention, 2021).

Fortunately, children recover well after a traumatic event. Unfortunately, some go on to develop PTSD that stays with them for months, years, or a lifetime. Recently, it has been discovered that children start to develop PTSD when they have trouble processing their trauma and perceive their symptoms as being extremely wrong signs (Watts et al., 2021). According to some research, PTSD often arises starting in early childhood, and although most children can recover independently from traumatic events, the individuals that cannot are those who develop persisting PTSD in their later lives. Hence, Watts et al.'s study was done to determine why some children have significant traumatic stress symptoms after trauma while others do not. The study also explored why some children recover without treatment while it takes other children a lot of time and effort to get treated and they go on to experience more persistent problems related to their PTSD (Watts et al., 2021). The research team worked with 396 college students to identify their childhood trauma history, cognitive processing, and PTSD experiences. The participants indicated trauma arising from car crashes, assaults, dog attacks, and other medical emergencies (Watts et al., 2021). Self-report surveys were used to assess for PTSD between two and four weeks following their trauma and again after two months. The research team also took into consideration patient coping mechanisms and how closely their maladaptive thoughts aligned with their inner schemas, meaning their perceptions of their own identities (Watts et al., 2021).

The research findings were telling. There was a high positive correlation between childhood emotional maltreatment and subsequent PTSD diagnosis, but this was largely mediated by intrusive rumination as an intervening variable. The results from the study showed that PTSD symptoms are fairly common early on following a childhood traumatic event, especially between two and four weeks following the trauma. These initial reactions and symptoms of PTSD are driven by high levels of fear and confusion during the trauma (Watts et al., 2021). The results also showed that the centrality of the event and intrusive rumination significantly affected the PTSD symptoms and recurrence. Given the deleterious effects of childhood emotional maltreatment, targeted intervention is required to treat PTSD, including through Narrative Therapy and Acceptance and Commitment Therapy. Furthermore, the fact that rumination is a significantly related causal factor for PTSD suggests that the researchers' results may be even more significant since self-report participants are likely to minimize or deny the severity of their experiences (Watts et al., 2021). Therefore, the study suggests that children who do not cope well with their trauma and cannot process traumatic events go on to develop PTSD after ruminating over their trauma. In turn, this may cause children to relive the traumatic experience and can negatively impact the emotional well-being of a child.

Luckily, there are many ways that PTSD can be treated in a child. Treatment depends on the individual child's symptoms, age, general health, and how severe the condition is (Stanford Children's Health, n.d.). PTSD has a high success rate if diagnosed early, since the sooner PTSD is diagnosed the more stability the child will gain and enhance their normal development (Stanford Children's Health, n.d.). Treatments include cognitive therapy whereby a child learns skills to handle his or her anxiety and to master the situation that led to the PTSD. Additionally, through pharmacotherapy, medicines for depression or anxiety can aid the children feel calmer. The recovery path from PTSD varies from child to child. Some children recover within six months whereas some take much longer, and this is due to the fact that recovery depends on the child's inner strengths, coping skills, and the ability to bounce back. It is also affected by the level of family support as parents and friends play a vital role throughout the process of treatment (Stanford Children's Health, n.d.). Parents and legal guardians should teach their children that it is completely alright to say no to someone who tries to touch their body inappropriately and make them feel uncomfortable. They should encourage their children to attend prevention programs in community or local school systems in order to prevent their child from experiencing any traumatic event and preventing PTSD from developing in their child (Stanford Children's Health, n.d.).

PTSD is prevalent among children, but it is the most common among adults, specifically adults who are not elderly and are younger than 65 years old (Naismith et al., 2024). According to a comprehensive study conducted to examine the combined effect of gender and age on PTSD, it was found that men and women differed in lifespan distribution of PTSD and the highest prevalence of PTSD was seen in the early 40s for men and the early 50s for women (Naismith et al., 2024). Women seem to have an overall twofold higher PTSD prevalence than men. This higher prevalence is because women have a higher chance of experiencing a traumatic event compared to men. Hence, adult women are twice as likely as men to develop PTSD during their lifetime (Naismith et al., 2024). Results from another study done on PTSD and its association with age group and gender showed that the highest rates of PTSD prevalence among both men and women are between the ages of 18 and 24 years and lowest among older age groups because some evidence points to the fact that potentially traumatic events, as well as the risk of developing PTSD are the same in adolescents and adults (Naismith et al., 2024). Moreover, it has been noticed that the elderly, aged 60 or older are the least likely to be diagnosed with PTSD among all three age groups since the tendency of PTSD prevalence rates declining from a young age to old age follows a linear decrease (Naismith et al., 2024). With increasing age, the risk of developing PTSD declines significantly especially in the elderly.

The symptoms that adults aged 18 to 59 and elderly aged 60 or older experience the same kind of symptoms of PTSD which include replaying intrusive memories about the traumatic event repeatedly again in their heads, avoiding thinking or talking about the event and avoiding places and activity or people that remind of the traumatic event, developing negative changes in thinking and mood such as negative thoughts about oneself, hopelessness, difficulty maintaining relationships, feeling detached from the world, feeling emotionally numb, lack of interest in all activities, sleeping issues, emotional and physical distress, suicidal thoughts, and overwhelming guilt and shame (Byllesby and Palmieri, 2023). These symptoms are extremely serious, and the sooner people receive treatment, the better. Fortunately, there are many useful resources that provide support to adults and elderly struggling with PTSD and help them throughout their treatment. It is best for the patient to stay in a positive social circle, talk to their doctor and therapist, and get medications that might be able to help the patients both mentally and physically.

Generally, findings from various studies show that people in their late teenage years to late adulthood are vulnerable to PTSD, with women most vulnerable during middle age and men being most vulnerable during late adulthood (Naismith et al., 2024). PTSD is a dangerous condition, and no one deserves to go through it, but unfortunately, there are crimes, natural disasters, and accidents that occur that cannot be controlled or prevented by humans. PTSD can develop in anyone whether it be a child, an adult, or an elderly person and it depends on the individual's circumstances and personal characteristics in terms of how they cope with PTSD. It is not easy for everyone to forget about a traumatic event and move on. Therefore, the best way to prevent anyone from going through PTSD is to spread awareness and organize events and workshops that teach people about PTSD. People should also be taught how to cope with it as well as how to stay strong mentally and practice resilience which aids an individual's ability to take something positive from adversity (Dodd et al., 2020). It is important to help people prevent PTSD since it is a condition that can affect anyone and at any age.

REFERENCES

Brooks, S. K, and N. Greenberg. "Recurrence of Post-Traumatic Stress Disorder: Systematic Review of Definitions, Prevalence and Predictors." *BMC Psychiatry* 24, no. 1: 1–37, 2024. https://doi:10.1186/s12888-023-05460-x

Brouzos, A., E. Vatkali, D. Mavridis, S. P. Vassilopoulos, and V. C. Baourda. "Psychoeducation for Adults with Post-Traumatic Stress Symptomatology: A Systematic Review and Meta-Analysis." *Journal of Contemporary Psychotherapy: On the Cutting Edge of Modern Developments in Psychotherapy* 52, no. 2: 155–64, 2022. https://doi:10.1007/s10879-021-09526-3

Byllesby, B. M., and P. A. Palmieri. "A Bifactor Model of General and Specific PTSD Symptom Change During Treatment." *Assessment* 30, no. 8: 2595–2604, 2023. https://doi:10.1177/10731911231156646

Centers for Disease Control and Prevention. "Post-Traumatic Stress Disorder in Children." Centers for Disease Control and Prevention, 2021. https://www.cdc.gov/childrensmentalhealth/ptsd.html

Dodd, C. G., R. M. Hill, L. M. Alvis, E. E. Rooney, C. M. Layne, T. Logsdon, I. N. Sandler, and J. B. Kaplow. "Initial Validation and Measurement Invariance of the Active Inhibition Scale Among

Traumatized and Grieving Youth." *Journal of Traumatic Stress* 33, no. 5: 843–49, October 2020. https://doi:10.1002/jts.22529

Li, J., L. Gao, R. Bao, R. Ji, Q. He, W. Zhang, X. Tang, and Z. Qu. "Comparative Efficacy for Different Age Groups of Psychological or Psychosocial Treatments on Post-Traumatic Stress Disorder: Protocol for Systematic Review, Meta-Analysis and Meta-Regression Analysis." *BMJ Open* 13, no. 1: e066569, 2023. https://doi:10.1136/bmjopen-2022-066569

Naismith, I., K. Ripoll-Nuñez, and G. Baquero Henao. "Depression, Anxiety, and Posttraumatic Stress Disorder Following Intimate Partner Violence: The Role of Self-Criticism, Guilt, and Gender Beliefs." *Violence Against Women* 30, nos. 3/4: 791–811, December 2024. https://doi:10.1177/10778012221142917

Stanford Children's Health. "Posttraumatic Stress Disorder (PTSD) in Children." n.d. https://www. stanfordchildrens.org/en/topic/default?id=post-traumatic-stress-disorder-in-children-90-P02579

Watts, J., M. Leeman, D. O'Sullivan, J. Castleberry, and G. Baniya. "Childhood Emotional Maltreatment and Post-Traumatic Stress Disorder in the Context of Centrality of the Event and Intrusive Rumination." *Rehabilitation Counseling Bulletin* 64, no. 2: 108–17, January 2021. https://doi:10.1177/0034355220925889

Zai, C. C., S. Y. Cheema, G. C. Zai, A. K. Tiwari, and J. L. Kennedy. "Post-Traumatic Stress Disorder in the Canadian Longitudinal Study on Aging: A Genome-Wide Association Study." *Journal of Psychiatric Research* 154: 209–218, October 2022. https://doi:10.1016/j.jpsychires.2022.07.049

Zaragoza Scherman, A., S. Salgado, Z. Shao, and D. Berntsen. "Younger Adults Report More Distress and Less Well-Being: A Cross-Cultural Study of Event Centrality, Depression, Posttraumatic Stress Disorder and Life Satisfaction." *Applied Cognitive Psychology* 34, no. 5: 1180–96, 2020. https://doi:10.1002/acp.3707

CHAPTER 11

TREATMENTS

There are many considerations for treating PTSD from different types of therapies to medical treatments, to dietary and lifestyle changes. Learning about the possible avenues of support and treatment is helpful for anyone both suffering with PTSD and looking to help those suffering with PTSD. The following is a brief overview of many different avenues for PTSD treatment.

COGNITIVE THERAPY

According to past and current research, the most effective method of physiological treatment is cognitive therapy. Cognitive therapy focuses on how trauma affects personal thoughts and beliefs. This therapy gathers an understanding of how the individual views themselves, people around them, and the world in general. The central aspect of cognitive therapy is based upon how the way we think affects the way in which we express our emotions ("Cognitive Processing Therapy," n.d.). Cognitive therapy uses this to alter the negative self-opinion. The primary goal is for PTSD sufferers to learn how to become aware of themselves and for clinicians to effectively be a part of the treatment. The first step is for the patient to understand how they personally perceive their surroundings, themselves, and how the trauma has changed their perspectives. After learning about a patient's perspectives, the clinician will then figure out how to change the mindset. The client should then know how to differentiate what is imagined and what is real.

It is helpful for patients to write down their thoughts so that their thoughts can be organized and be an external outlet for their feelings along with providing a record for the clinician. One of the complaints against cognitive therapy is that it does not directly improve the lives of the patients. This therapy provides the possibility for adjustment. By becoming self-aware and conscious of thoughts, the individuals receiving therapy can change their actions through changing the way they think—actions come from thoughts. With dedication to cognitive therapy, the patient can learn to live a more positive lifestyle and deal with the after-effects of the trauma.

COMPLEMENTARY AND ALTERNATIVE METHODS (CAM)

Although posttraumatic stress disorder is clinically classified as a psychological disorder, it can be treated with alternative methods. Another option is complementary and alternative methods (CAM). This means the patient will have two methods of treatment ongoing simultaneously. The conventional method is medication and can be accompanied by, but is not limited to meditation, hypnosis, massage, and relaxation ("Complementary and Alternative Medicine," 2023). Most sufferers of PTSD try conventional methods of treatment first prior to complementary treatment. Although complementary techniques have been proven to result in positive results in the patient, it is important to seek proper professional help from a clinician. The best results for overcoming PTSD come from following CAM, which is using conventional and alternative methods together.

PHYSICAL ACTIVITY

Participating in as much physical activity as possible provides many benefits; it encourages a healthy lifestyle and body. Exercise and physical movement have been shown to significantly reduce stress and depression symptoms. It can be as simple as walking outside, performing tasks or chores, going to the gym, participating in sports, or taking weekly exercise classes. Sufferers tend to isolate themselves inside, and physical activity encourages them to leave their comfort zone and go outside. One study was able to prove improvement of PTSD symptoms with physical exercise, which improves further with a mixed exercise routine rather than just one form of exercise (Jadhakhan et al., 2022). Although exercise is a good step toward establishing a positive outlook and rein-troduction to social interaction, it does not guarantee a healthy mental state. Yoga and Tai Chi are calming activities that have the ability to help patients calm their minds and compose their feelings. These exercises are based on control and balance and aid in connecting the mind and body. Doing yoga and Tai Chi in a natural outdoor environment may further amplify its benefits.

NUTRITION AND DIET

Maintaining a healthy diet and nutrition is often overlooked by PTSD sufferers. A poor nutritional diet, such as too much fatty food, lack of carbohydrates, and insufficient fruits and vegetables, will lead to consti-pation and low energy levels. This intensifies the symptoms.

When a PTSD victim is suffering from depression, health and nutrition is not on their minds. Preparing proper meals can be an overwhelming chore. It is not uncommon for patients to turn to fast food and unhealthy alternatives. Foods with high sugar and fat causes emotions to fluctuate greatly and contribute to low-energy levels and fatigue. Although patients may argue that healthy food is more time-consuming and less financially efficient, a regular intake of vitamins and mineral supplements can help solve this. Some recommended nutra-ceuticals include Vitamin D, folate, antioxidants, magnesium, omega-3 fatty acids, vitamin B6, vitamin B9, vitamin B12, and phospholipid sup-plements which can supply essential nutrition for those suffering with mental health conditions and help to improve neurotransmitter activity and cognitive abilities within the brain (Korn, 2022). It is an effective method of ensuring patients receive most of the vitamins they need in their bodies. That being said, the best method is still to prepare and eat healthy foods.

BREATHING RELAXATION

Due to the extreme feelings of anxiousness, sadness, anger, and help-lessness, PTSD sufferers may have headaches, stomachaches, irregular bowel movements, muscle aches, poor sleep habits, and constant states of fatigue. These are reactions our bodies have to large amounts of stress. Experiencing these negative emotions over a period of time takes a toll on our bodies physiologically. Relaxation is necessary for recovery. Not only does a PTSD victim need rest, but also people involved with the victim's recovery process need to take time to rest. Caretakers, family, and friends cannot care for someone else if they are exhausted. Breathing-based relaxation is a helpful technique for everyone involved. When an individual is stressed or hyperaroused, physiologically, the heart rate increases, and breathing will also become faster and sharper. This can be painful to experience. By controlling how the breaths are taken, patients can become calmer and more focused. An article that appeared on the Othership site lists three types of breathing exercises, which are by no means exhaustive, but still a great start for anyone looking to try different ways of breathing to calm themselves. These exercises are called "biodynamic breathwork," "holotropic breathwork," and "Win Hof breathwork method" ("Breathwork for Healing Trauma," 2021). These exercises all combine different forms of breathing and thought practice to focus the mind and relax the body. Once the body begins to relax, breathing will be steady, and there will be a lower oxygen level in the bloodstream and a slower heart rate. The great thing about these breathing exercises is that they can be used almost anytime, and almost anywhere, allowing for instant relief of heightened emotions or hyperarousal.

HYPNOSIS

Over the years, hypnosis has been known as a form of pseudoscience and has become extremely popular. Patients who undergo hypnosis are brought into a deep state of relaxation. Therapists offer patients one or two internal suggestions in the scenario of trauma that offer the possibility to adjust the result or perspective of the outcome, such as making a different decision or taking a third-person stance (Lemig, 2022). Before the end of a session, the clients are encouraged and led toward positive thoughts so that they feel secure and can relax prior to returning to reality as they wake up. Hypnosis is not effective for all clients depending on the severity of the trauma or if the client is resistant. When hypnosis is a method of treatment being used, it should not be the sole treatment a patient is receiving.

ANIMAL THERAPY

More recently, animals have been used as therapeutic helpers with mental health conditions including PTSD. The notion of having responsibility of taking care of another living being compels a pet owner to also take care of themselves. As pet owners, they are in an interdependent relationship. Pets can become part of the victim's support system by providing comfort and can be more reliable than the people around the individual.

In the past few years there has been an increase in the number of programs encouraging animal therapy. There are available therapy sessions for PTSD sufferers to interact with animals for short periods of time. This aids in the transition of caring for a pet; the patients are not pressured into taking immediate responsibility for their pet. Encouraged interactions between patients and animals and helped decrease the likelihood of severe depression. Taking care of a pet requires a schedule including many feedings, walking, and sleeping. There are also opportunities for service dogs in respect to PTSD, where the dogs are trained to help the owner with any stressors or tasks. Also, because they are service dogs, they can accompany the sufferer to almost any facility ("Dogs and PTSD," n.d.).

The schedule of pet care also helps to foster an organized lifestyle and encourages more physical movement. For example, having a dog will encourage the owner to go outside to walk their dog. A dog will also encourage the owner to wake up at a designated time. Although this increases the tasks and responsibilities required of their owners, pets are loyal and create a loving environment for recovery. PTSD pet owners don't need to worry about acceptance or judgment. For patients considering animal therapy, pets should not be simply given, rather pets and owners should choose each other.

MEDICATIONS

Medical intervention is one of the most commonly used methods of treatment for PTSD. There are medications that can be very effective in dealing with the symptoms of PTSD. One study concluded the efficacy of SSRIs in treating PTSD as first-line drugs for treating the illness, where 58% of the test subjects had improved symptoms of PTSD while using SSRI medications (Williams et al., 2022). Other medications include antidepressants, prazosin, novel antipsychotics, and other medications for sleep disturbance. Generally, medication tends to produce smaller improvement results than the previously mentioned therapies, but it is a choice of treatment that is often chosen.

There are two major advantages to the use of medication in treating PTSD. First, it requires minimal intervention after the initial diagnosis. Second, medication produces immediate improvements to PTSD conditions and is also why many patients start medical treatment after diagnosis. Immediate improvements are helpful for patients in continuing their regular routines and lifestyles. Despite the advantages, there are limitations. There can be significant side effects and risks. Although not all patients are necessarily susceptible to any or all side effects, it is a reason why some choose not to receive this method of treatment. There is also no one-size-fits-all treatment. Although one drug may work for one person, it does not necessarily work for another, even within the same family. The process of introducing medication is a trial-and-error sort of process with regular reports to medical professionals to ensure that the drugs are working as indicated. It is also worth noting that once patients are no longer using the medication, the symptoms of PTSD resume. Medication needs to be taken consistently.

The other options for therapy for PTSD victims are long-term investments toward improvement in behavior and symptoms. The psychotherapies rely instead on helping patients develop coping mechanisms and trigger recognitions which results in more independence and self-reliance for dealing with their conditions.

REFERENCES

"Breathwork for Healing Trauma: 3 Popular Techniques + Benefits." Othership, October 17, 2021. https://www.othership.us/resources/breathwork-for-healing-trauma

"Cognitive Processing Therapy (CPT) for PTSD." U.S. Department of Veterans Affairs, n.d. https://www.ptsd.va.gov/understand_tx/cognitive_processing.asp

"Complementary and Alternative Medicine." National Cancer Institute, June 12, 2023. https://www.cancer.gov/about-cancer/treatment/cam

"Dogs and PTSD." U.S. Department of Veterans Affairs, n.d. https://www.ptsd.va.gov/gethelp/dogs_ptsd.asp

Jadhakhan, F., N. Lambert, N. Middlebrook, D. W. Evans, and D. Falla. "Is Exercise/Physical Activity Effective at Reducing Symptoms of Post-Traumatic Stress Disorder in Adults—a Systematic Review." Frontiers in *Psychology* 13, August 12, 2022. https://doi.org/10.3389/fpsyg.2022.943479

Korn, L. "Exploring Integrative Medicine and Nutrition for PTSD." *Psychiatric Times*, October 21, 2022https://www.psychiatrictimes.com/view/exploring-integrative-medicine-and-nutrition-for-ptsd

Lemig, C. "Hypnosis for PTSD: How It Works, Effectiveness, & Examples." Choosing Therapy, May 17, 2022. https://www.choosingtherapy.com/hypnosis-for-ptsd/

Williams, T., N. J. Phillips, D. J. Stein, and J. C. Ipser. "Pharmacotherapy for Post Traumatic Stress Disorder (PTSD)." Cochrane Database of Systematic Reviews 2022, no. 3, March 2, 2022. https://doi.org/10.1002/14651858.cd002795.pub3

CHAPTER 12

OTHER RISKS (COMORBIDITY)

Posttraumatic stress disorder occurs after an individual has experienced trauma. During the trauma, the victim's fear is triggered, and the body reacts with a fight-or-flight response. After the physiological response, those affected by PTSD have difficulties returning to a regular physiological state after their ability to do so has been changed. PTSD individuals are in a constant state of stress and fear, even after the trauma has passed. As a result of this increased state of arousal, these victims of PTSD experience multiple symptoms. In addition, a majority of these individuals will begin to suffer from other medical or physical illnesses (Qassem et al., 2020). When an individual is experiencing two or more medical conditions at the same time, it is known as comorbidity. The diagnosis of comorbidity is the existence of two or more disorders at the same time within one person. This does not mean that the initial signs of both disorders have to appear at the same time. It is possible for one condition to start and be followed by one of more other disorders. As long as the symptoms of the two disorders are overlapping, it is considered to be comorbid. Comorbidity with PTSD has been found to reach 78.5% of all PTSD cases (Qassem et al., 2020). If an individual has two disorders, they are comorbid. Once the symptoms of one condition stops, however, the individual is no longer comorbid. Victims of posttraumatic stress disorder often also have depression, suicidal thoughts, and behaviors, and tend to abuse substances.

DEPRESSION

Depression is known by multiple names in the medical world, but it is most commonly identified as major depression, major depressive disorder, and clinical depression. Most people identify depression as being sad, blue, miserable, unhappy, or "down in the dumps." Many individuals do not realize the seriousness and consequences that come with depression because the symptoms are similar to feelings that they may have felt at one time or another. Depression has been marked as the most condition to coexist with PTSD (Qassem et al., 2020). The medical field defines *depression* as a condition that causes an individual to feel persistent sadness, loss, anger, frustration, and a loss of interest in their own everyday life. Depression affects victims on a physical level ("What Is Depression?" 2020). Mental disorders do not have the same effect on everyone. Every person's brain is structured differently; it is why everyone deals with trauma differently and responds to treatment differently. Various reactions also occur because of the victim's experiences, which may include past trauma. There are eight recognized depressive disorders within the *DSM-V* that highlight the different ways in which people experience states of depression (*DSM-V*, 2022). While many of these disorders feature the aforementioned feelings associated with a deeper sense of sadness, it is a major depressive disorder that is most often found to be comorbid with PTSD. According to studies, 48% of PTSD cases were comorbid with major depression (Qassem et al., 2020). The added similarities between major depression criterion and those of PTSD listed within the *DSM-V* also lead to confusion in diagnosis. For example, both criterion C and D for PTSD which discuss avoidance behavior and negative changes in mood can be associated with the onset of a major depressive disorder which lists similar criterion (*DSM-V*, 2022). This area of overlap can sometimes be cause for confusion and is a great way to highlight why it is so important to be aware of and search for comorbidity within patients with PTSD.

SUBSTANCE ABUSE

Substance abuse has been defined in the medical world as the continuous use of harmful substances for the intention of altering mood and mental state. Other definitions also state drug abuse as a person's use of illicit drugs or over-the-counter drugs. These drugs are used for a purpose other than that which is its original intention, usually in extreme quantities. It has become difficult to correctly identify all of the new substances that are being abused. It is not just illegal drugs that are being abused. Today, the abuse has extended to prescription drugs and even mouthwash. Studies have found that people who suffer with PTSD are more likely to develop a substance abuse disorder than those who do not have PTSD (Dell'Aquila and Berle, 2023). The addiction can start with a casual or social situation and the user becomes attached to the effects the substance can give. For PTSD sufferers who also have addictions, their substance abuse stems from wanting to avoid the feelings of fear and pain from the trauma (Dell'Aquila and Berle, 2023). Intense anxiety, intrusive memories, and flashbacks are experienced from day-to-day life. Substance abuse is a way for sufferers to gain a small measure of control over their own lives, however brief that may be. In their attempts to gain control, they lose even more control than before as substance abuse takes over. Studies have shown that over 30% of those genetically predisposed to PTSD are also predisposed to alcohol abuse disorder (Hawn et al., 2020). This shows the high likelihood of developing concurrent problems with both PTSD and substance abuse. Additionally, the comorbidity rates of 30%–50% for alcohol use disorder and PTSD further highlight the significance of treating disorders as they arise before comorbidity exacerbates the conditions (Hawn et al., 2020). Continuous usage of substances as a means of escape increases their dependence on the substances. Instead of avoiding fear and anxiety, it actually worsens. PTSD and substance abuse is a vicious cycle and becomes extremely challenging for the victim to leave behind.

When seeking treatment for the co-occurring disorders of PTSD and addiction, the most effective way to recover is to seek intensive support from psychiatric professionals and having an extremely strong support system of friends and family. Although symptoms can be managed through professional assistance, many individuals choose not to seek treatment from the guilt and shame they feel through their conditions. A lot of their guilt rises from the belief that they could have done something or something differently to prevent their trauma. The victims feel helpless for the inability to move on from the trauma.

Many sufferers feel guilty because of their lack of understanding about how their condition affects them. Guilt prevents a PTSD victim from seeking proper treatment and attempting to self-medicate. Through substance abuse, their willingness to seek professional help decreases. By having a proper support system in place, family and friends can encourage the individual to seek proper treatment and complete the treatment process.

SUICIDAL THOUGHTS AND BEHAVIORS

Sufferers of PTSD are very likely to have suicidal thoughts and behaviors due to not only having to deal with symptoms, but also comorbidity. Suicide has been defined in the medical field as a person harming themselves with the intention of taking his or her own life. In normal circumstances of suicide, individuals take their own life as a reaction to stressful life situations or events. Suicidal thoughts can be the result of being unable to cope with an intense internal feeling, or emotions brought on by a traumatic event. These causes of suicide are very similar to the symptoms that are associated with posttraumatic stress disorder.

When a PTSD victim becomes too overwhelmed by emotions such as fear and anxiety, they turn to other behaviors in order to cope. The commonness of comorbidity increases the likelihood for the victim to turn to suicide. When they feel that they can no longer deal with their issues every day of their life suicide becomes a choice they may take.

Although PTSD is difficult to deal with on its own, having it co-occur with another condition makes it even more challenging but not impossible. In cases where PTSD has led to other disorders it is essential that the victim seeks professional help immediately. In addition, those around the victim need to support them, because without the encouragement and reinforcement the probability of recovery falls significantly. In a best-case scenario, the victim will choose to deal with their PTSD before it reaches the point of bringing on other conditions. If the worst happens, the most important thing to do is deal with each of the conditions from the most severe to least. This is an essential step to follow because it eliminates the most immediate problem first, allowing the individual to have time to adjust and deal with their other issues, in a slower stride.

REFERENCES

Dell'Aquila, A., and D. Berle. "Predictors of Alcohol and Substance Use among People with Post-Traumatic Stress Disorder (PTSD): Findings from the NESARC-III Study." *Social Psychiatry and Psychiatric Epidemiology* 58, no. 10: 1509–22, May 3, 2023. https://doi.org/10.1007/s00127-023-02472-6

Hawn, S. E., S. E. Cusack, and A. B. Amstadter. "A Systematic Review of the Self-Medication Hypothesis in the Context of Posttraumatic Stress Disorder and Comorbid Problematic Alcohol Use." *Journal of Traumatic Stress* 33, no. 5: 699–708, June 9, 2020. https://doi.org/10.1002/jts.22521

Qassem, T., D. Aly-ElGabry, A. Alzarouni, K. Abdel-Aziz, and D. Arnone. "Psychiatric Co-Morbidities in Post-Traumatic Stress Disorder: Detailed Findings from the Adult Psychiatric Morbidity Survey in the English Population." *Psychiatric Quarterly* 92, no. 1: 321–30, July 23, 2020. https://doi.org/10.1007/s11126-020-09797-4

"What Is Depression?" Psychiatry.org, October 2020. https://www.psychiatry.org/patients-families/depression/what-is-depression

13

WHAT IS STILL UNKNOWN?

osttraumatic stress disorder (PTSD) is a psychiatric disorder which has the ability to occur in individuals who have witnessed a traumatic event (Bhandari, 2022). The traumatic event can be defined with many examples such as sexual violence, an accident, or a natural disaster. Additionally, any individual is capable of developing PTSD, whether it be through their occupation or family. For instance, multiple studies have shown, out of 60,000 Iraq and Afghanistan veterans, 13.5% developed PTSD, whereas others had a 20%–30% chance of developing it (U.S. Department of Veteran Affairs, 2021). Along with that, PTSD can also occur indirectly. In essence, families of victims have the possibility of becoming diagnosed with PTSD (Bhandari, 2022). This is because individuals tend to develop a sense of helplessness, fear, and guilt. Although these emotions are experienced by every human being, people with PTSD have a long-lasting effect from them; they are unable to overcome their emotions as well as their feelings have the possibility of becoming strong overtime.

For example, some of the symptoms of PTSD include the person reliving the event, avoiding certain places, having an intense physical and/ or emotional reaction, and increasing their pessimistic cognition. Moreover, PTSD has the capability of developing at any age. Statistically, in the United States, six out of one hundred people can develop PTSD (U.S. Department of Veteran Affairs, 2023). Additionally, in adults, 10% of women and 4% of men develop PTSD in the United States, whereas in teens and children, 14% of girls and 6% of boys develop PTSD.

Hence, due to the number of cases each year, medications and psycho-therapy have been used as treatments for PTSD. For medications, doc-tors prescribe certain antidepressants or blood pressure medicines to control various symptoms and emotions. As for psychotherapy, individ-uals with PTSD attend sessions for family therapy, group therapy, psy-chodynamic therapy, or eye desensitization and reprocessing (EMDR). Nonetheless, every individual with PTSD experiences different trau-mas and feelings. Hence, every one of these individuals require a spe-cific type of treatment. Although these treatments have the potential to fully cure an individual, there are many cases where they fail to do so. In addition, many people are self-stigmatized or pressured by others to not report their conditions, which leads to individuals living with PTSD their whole life. Although there is a lot of known information about PTSD, a lot of things are still unknown. Thus, this chapter would focus on what we do not know about posttraumatic stress disorder.

As discussed, every case of PTSD stems from a unique traumatic experience and therefore has differences in the types of symptoms, the extent of their disorder, and some other factors which also affect the treatment they are supposed to receive. In 1969, one of the research-ers in the APA Society of Clinical Psychology, named Gordon L. Paul, proposed a question asking the specific type of treatment necessary to treat a specific problem with a specific person, wondering more about under what conditions this sort of treatment might arise (Hayes et. al., 2020). Even with the advancements in technology and research, this question still remains unanswered. Treatments suggested for PTSD for a specific individual requires an accurate diagnosis but the diagnostic systems, such as *Diagnostic and Statistical Manual of Mental Disorders (DSM)* and *International Classification of Disease (ICD)*, do not con-sider etiology, social networks, family affairs, intrapsychic conflicts, and ego strengths as important factors (Bovin et al., 2021).

Unfortunately, a specific treatment for a specific individual remains unknown. For instance, according to the *DSM* diagnosis, there is a fixed criteria that one needs to fall under in order to be diagnosed with PTSD (Bovin et. al., 2021). Although the system is effective in diagnosing, it fails to provide the correct treatment for the patient. In past years, a lot of models have been introduced which may help therapists decide on a particular process to treat a patient. For example, in 1990, Beutler and Clarkin developed a model which considered the patient, the therapist, the therapeutic factors, and the therapy's overtime process (Nguyen et al, 2023). Nonetheless, the model failed to provide satisfying results, hence, to this day, an accepted model, which can accurately guide researchers to choose relevant and required patient variables, does not exist. Therefore, the question about how to approach specific client treatment has remained unanswered to date. Since PTSD is an extremely complicated disorder, varying from person to person, it is difficult to develop and find a satisfying model (or answer) which can be used to treat patients. Nonetheless, research continues to advance further, thus, potentially in the future, an answer to this question can be expected.

In order to evaluate and investigate PTSD, it is crucial to know what caused it to happen in the first place. Despite the vast amount of research done on PTSD however, its exact causation remains unknown. Nonetheless, researchers have taken into account the extent at which a particular factor might develop PTSD in an individual. The big unanswerable question with PTSD is how far genetic and environmental factors can be linked with the onset of PTSD. Heritability explains the ability to pass genetic material from parents to offspring. Questions concerning the heritability of mental health conditions has been an ongoing question in science for some time. In the field of genetics, "the G-by-E effect," or rather the correlation between genetic (G) and environment(E) factors in determining the heritability of mental health conditions, refers to the complexity of determining the cross-contamination of genetic versus environmental factors (Zhang, H. et al., 2022). For example, consider two people who might be genetically predisposed to developing PTSD. If only one of those two people experiences trauma, then only that one person is likely to develop PTSD. Therefore, there needs to be a consideration of both genetic and environmental factors, always. The imagined ideal set of information for analyzing environmental versus genetic factors in human diseases would include complete genetic details for a large quantity of people, complete phenotypic profiles for all people involved, and a thorough documentation of all exterior environmental experiences (Zhang, H. et al., 2022). Realistically, achieving such a thorough collection of the aforementioned data proves to be an insurmountable task. Because of this, current studies rely on simple, cheaper, datasets, and math that can significantly simplify assumptions which allows inference where data is incomplete. There are three such groups of approaches in existing research used to discern this type of information, called "Twin Studies," "Pedigree Studies," and "'Whole-Genome Sequences and Genetic Association Studies" (Zhang, H. et al., 2022). Because each type of study allows for some simplification in the math, each study results in some sort of bias. For example, in twin studies, all factors displayed between both twins is assumed to be genetic, while pedigree studies included limited genetic and environmental data that might offer more balance in "the G-by-E effect," but still remains woefully lacking in data (Zhang, H et al., 2022). High values of hc^2 reveal that two parents in a nuclear family setting are often more similar both genetically and environmentally than initially expected. This might indicate that both parents had similar exposures leading to their PTSD, rather than specifically genetic factors (Zhang, H. et al., 2022). These findings, unfortunately, remain largely inconclusive because of the theoretical limitations set forth by the type of research. Although lacking clarity in long-term studies, there have been advancements made in the understanding of genetic factors with regard to PTSD. For example, studies have revealed a relationship between ADCYAP1R1 polymorphism and PTSD. Though highly contested in the scientific field, some associations have been made to suggest the C allele results in a higher potential for developing PTSD (Zhang, J. et al., 2022). Such results, however, remain highly inconsistent, potentially due to a study method which only measures the PTSD symptoms of a patient one time (Zhang, J. et al., 2022). Future studies involving multiple measurements of PTSD symptoms throughout the study phase might provide more concrete information about the relationship between ADCYAP1R1 and PTSD. Out of 1, 017 children and adolescent survivors of the Wenchuan earthquake in 2008, girls between 2.5 years and 4.5 years after the disaster were connected with the gene-environment effects of the ADCYAP1R1 polymorphism rs2267735 (Zhang, J. et al., 2022). Findings such as these confirm that there can be important genetic factors which play a role in the onset and course of PTSD symptoms in patients. Despite such research, there is still little known about the long-term development of PTSD after the initial experience of trauma. Thus, at this time it is determined that our initial question of whether PTSD develops due to environmental and/or genetic factors cannot be definitively addressed without the expensive, and near impossible to achieve. Further research, however, needs to be conducted in order to understand the main cause of PTSD. Although researchers have investigated several factors behind why an individual would have a higher chance of developing PTSD as compared to others, the exact source remains unknown.

Adding on to the types of factors that might trigger PTSD, researchers have investigated the effects of gun violence, riots, and revolutions on PTSD development. It is crucial to consider that it is not required for an individual to experience a traumatic event directly in order to develop PTSD. Nonetheless, people who do get directly exposed to the events, such as arson, a serious physical injury, and looting, have a higher chance of developing PTSD (Ni et al., 2020). Furthermore, people who are exposed to violence through close proximity, media exposure, and personal attack, are also at risk of developing PTSD. Nonetheless, there is not enough research conducted behind the effects of gun violence on PTSD; it is unknown if PTSD has a correlation with attitudes toward guns and gun violence. Especially in the United States, people continue to have exposure to gun violence which is considered as one of the most traumatic events that can cause PTSD. According to research, carrying a gun might be one of the consequences of PTSD. For instance, postwar veterans, who were diagnosed with PTSD, had a higher probability of owning a gun and using it to threaten others, as compared to veterans who did not have PTSD (Richman, 2020).

Furthermore, apart from postwar veterans, individuals who have experienced traumatic events such as a revolution, physical assault, robbery, and abduction, may use guns as a defense mechanism to protect themselves in order to prevent an event from repeating. Although PTSD causes individuals to become more aware of their surroundings, there is yet to be more research needed to examine the symptoms of PTSD when considering attitudes toward owning a gun and using it. Using the criteria of the *DSM-V*, individuals with PTSD are more likely to look out for danger, be paranoid, and have an exaggerated reaction, as compared to individuals without PTSD. Hence, carrying a weapon is one of the ways in which they can defend themselves. This also means that their reaction toward potential danger can cause harm to another individual. Along with that, it is necessary to consider that many postwar veterans with PTSD have a shock or a sense of horror when hearing a gunshot; what would be their reaction if the one firing the gun is themselves? Would they be hesitant or confident when firing it? Would having control over the gun change the way they react as compared to when someone else is firing it? Additionally, would their PTSD get triggered immediately or would the adrenaline overcome their reaction caused by PTSD? These questions are some of the examples as to why PTSD is a complex disorder. Undoubtedly, every individual has a difference in the type of traumatic event they experienced, the symptoms they displayed, and the reactions they show during a particular situation. Henceforth, researchers cannot have one specific answer behind what exactly causes PTSD.

PTSD is a disorder which affects all individuals no matter the age group. Hence, children are also one of the victims of PTSD. Whether it be neglect, abuse, or experiencing a natural disaster, children tend to become traumatized much more easily as compared to adults. Nonetheless, with increasing cases, there has been an increase in the amount of treatment options available for children to overcome PTSD (Substance Abuse and Mental Health Services Administration, 2023). Advancements in research have improved and increased the knowledge about PTSD in children and adolescents. Still, there are many factors that limit that knowledge leading to a lot of unknowns. The difference between *The International Classification of Diseases (ICD)* and the *Diagnostic Statistical Manual of Mental Disorders (DSM)* reveals a significant gap in the understanding, diagnosing, and treating of children with PTSD. For example, some studies found that *ICD-11* had a better fitting model by which to measure and diagnose PTSD in children across genders, and also found that children who met the criteria under the *DSM-V* were more likely to have comorbid diagnoses of anxiety and depression (Cloitre et al., 2020). Alternatively, in treatment-seeking samples, with a group of late adolescents to early adulthood patients with a history of abuse, the *ICD-11* involved a significant drop in the probability of being diagnosed with PTSD due to the sense of threat criterion (Cloitre et al., 2020). Though the *DSM-V* does not make the distinction of CPTSD, there are several child and adolescent studies which support the distinction in children. These studies determined that CPTSD groups revealed higher rates of childhood trauma, revealing the significant gaps between the *DSM-V* and the *ICD-11* when diagnosing and treating children (Cloitre et al., 2020). As a result of the glaring gap between the two foremost diagnostic tools for PTSD and other mental health conditions, further research should be done to assess the entire scope of mental health, and specifically PTSD, among youth, to develop a standard of diagnosis and treatment for children.

In conclusion, posttraumatic stress disorder (PTSD) is a psychiatric disorder which has the capability of developing at any stage of life through any traumatic event. Although there is a vast amount of information that is known about PTSD, many questions still remain unanswered. Due to the complexity of this disorder, a lot of features relating to PTSD are unknown to this day. As research behind PTSD continues, there is a possibility that, in the future, the unknowns would be known, questions would be answered, and hidden information behind PTSD would be revealed. Therefore, in the next chapter, the research that is being done currently, as well as the potential research that would be done in the future, will be discussed.

REFERENCES

Bhandari, S., Ed. "Posttraumatic Stress Disorder (PTSD): Symptoms, Diagnosis, Treatment." WebMD, August 31, 2022. https://www. webmd.com/mental-health/post-traumatic-stress-disorder

Bovin, M., A. Camden, and F. Weathers. "Literature on DSM-5 and I–D-11 - National Center for PTSD." U.S Department of Veterans Affairs, 2021. https://www.ptsd.va.gov/publications/rq_docs/V32N2.pdf

Cloitre, M., C. R. Brewin, E. Kazlauskas, B. Lueger-Schuster, T. Karatzias, P. Hyland, and M. Shevlin. "Commentary: The Need for Research on PTSD in Children and Adolescents—a Commentary on Elliot et al. (2020)." *Journal of Child Psychology and Psychiatry* 62, no. 3: 277–79, December 2, 2020. https://doi.org/10.1111/jcpp.13361

Hayes, S. C., S. G. Hofmann, and J. Ciarrochi. "A Process-Based Approach to Psychological Diagnosis and Treatment: The Conceptual and Treatment Utility of an Extended Evolutionary Meta Model." *Clinical Psychology Review* 82, December 2020. https://www.ncbi.nlm.nih.gov/pmc/articles/PMC7680437/

Nguyen, T., M. Bertoni, M. Charvat, and A. Gheytanchi. "Systematic Treatment Selection (STS): A Review and Future Directions.," ResearchGate, November 28, 2023. https://www.researchgate.net/publication/26459238_Systematic_Treatment_Selection_STS_A_Review_and_Future_Directions

Ni, M. Y., Y. Kim, I. McDowell, S. Wong, H. Qiu, I. O. Wong, S. Galea, and G. M. Leung. "Mental Health During and After Protests, Riots, and Revolutions: A Systematic Review." *Australian & New Zealand Journal of Psychiatry* 54, no. 3: 232–43, 2020. https://doi.org/10.1177/0004867419899165

"Recognizing and Treating Child Traumatic Stress." SAMHSA, August 3, 2023. https://www.samhsa.gov/child-trauma/recognizing-and-treating-child-traumatic-stress

Richman, M. "We're Here Anytime, Day or Night—24/7." Study: Veterans with PTSD More Likely to Have Justice-System Involvement Than Those Without." August 4, 2020. https://www.research.va.gov/currents/0820-Veterans-with-PTSD-more-likely-to-have-justice-system-involvement.cfm

Zhang, H., A. Khan, and A. Rzhetsky. "Gene-Environment Interactions Explain a Substantial Portion of Variability of Common Neuropsychiatric Disorders." *Cell Reports Medicine* 3, no. 9: 100736, September 6, 2022. https://doi.org/10.1016/j.xcrm.2022.100736

Zhang, J., G. Li, H. Yang, C. Cao, R. Fang, P. Liu, S. Luo, et al. "The Main Effect and Gene-Environment Interaction Effect of the ADCYAP1R1 Polymorphism RS2267735 on the Course of Posttraumatic Stress Disorder Symptoms—a Longitudinal Analysis." *Frontiers in Psychiatry* 13, October 28, 2022. https://doi.org/10.3389/fpsyt.2022.1032837

CHAPTER 14

CURRENT AND FUTURE RESEARCH

As described in previous chapters, posttraumatic stress disorder (PTSD) is a serious mental health disorder that can have devastating effects on a person's life if left untreated. While the condition has been around for thousands of years, it only came to be officially known as PTSD in 1980, when it was added to the American Psychological Association's *Diagnostic and Statistical Manual of Mental Disorders*—otherwise known as the *DSM* ("The Dangers of Untreated PTSD," n.d.). As such, the field of PTSD research is still relatively new. Nevertheless, the few decades of available research have led to a variety of treatments for PTSD, despite the vast number of questions that have yet to be answered.

This chapter aims to provide an overview of ongoing PTSD research, as well as the research that will likely be conducted in the coming years. An overview of current and future evidence-informed treatments will be provided. Along with that, factors—both lifestyle and genetic—that may affect a person's susceptibility to PTSD will be discussed. This will be tied into research about the neurobiological mechanisms of PTSD. Finally, there will be a discussion about the improvements that need to be made to the field of PTSD research—including those pertaining to research methods and funding.

TREATMENT

Based on research to date, the American Psychological Association (2020) strongly recommends that people experiencing PTSD seek out one of a few different treatments. These include cognitive behavioral Therapy (CBT), cognitive processing therapy (CPT), cognitive therapy, and prolonged exposure therapy (American Psychological Association, 2020). Each of the treatments involve a slight variation in timelines and methods, but each of their goals involve changing the way patients think about and process their trauma through regular, usually weekly, sessions with a therapist, either individually or in a group setting. CPT and cognitive therapy are both quite closely linked to CBT, which involves exploring the relationships between thoughts, feelings, and emotions, and leveraging these connections to change patterns that may be causing PTSD symptoms (American Psychological Association, 2020). Current research on PTSD treatments focuses on improvements and alternatives to these therapies, as well as the efficacy of various types of treatments for different types of traumas.

WRITTEN EXPOSURE THERAPY (WET)

This randomized noninferiority clinical trial aimed to evaluate the effectiveness of a five-session written exposure therapy (WET) compared to a more time-intensive ten-session cognitive processing therapy (CPT) in treating PTSD among active-duty service members. Carried out between August 2016 and October 2020, the research involved 169 predominantly Army participants, averaging 34 years of age, of whom 80.5% were male (Sloan et al., 2020). The primary objective was to determine whether WET was not inferior to CPT in reducing PTSD symptom severity, assessed using the Clinician-Administered PTSD Scale for DSM-5 (CAPS-5). Participants were randomly assigned to receive either WET (five weekly sessions) or CPT (twelve twice-weekly sessions). Evaluations were conducted at baseline and at ten, twenty, and thirty weeks postinitial treatment session, with PTSD symptom severity measured using CAPS-5. Noninferiority was defined as the difference between the two groups being below the upper bound of the 1-sided 95% confidence interval (CI), with a specified margin of ten points on the CAPS-5. Findings indicated that WET was not inferior to CPT, with a difference in outcome change between the treatment conditions of

3.96 points on the CAPS-5. The upper limit of the one-sided 95% CI consistently remained under ten points across all time points, ranging from 4.59 at week thirty to 6.81 at week ten. Additionally, participants in the WET group demonstrated higher completion rates of all treatment sessions compared to those in the CPT group. In conclusion, the study suggests that WET represents an effective and more efficient treatment alternative for service members with PTSD. Future research should concentrate on identifying factors influencing treatment outcomes to optimize the selection of suitable interventions for individuals grappling with PTSD (Sloan et al., 2020).

This research (Sloan et al., 2020) presents certain limitations. As expected, participants who withdrew prematurely were less inclined to attend subsequent assessments. Another potential drawback was the absence of long-term follow-up, preventing researchers from determining whether treatment effects endured beyond six months postintervention. Both WET and CPT significantly decreased PTSD symptom severity among service members to comparable extents, despite CPT requiring more time and resources. Generally, fewer individuals discontinued WET compared to CPT. The availability of a brief PTSD treatment is likely highly beneficial in military contexts, where operational duties may restrict treatment engagement. A notable observation in this study is the considerable variation in treatment outcomes among service members. A more comprehensive understanding of the factors influencing who benefits from PTSD treatment is a crucial area for further exploration in the field.

EXPOSURE THERAPY

Exposure therapy is classified as a behavioral intervention for PTSD as it addresses learned behaviors, particularly avoidance, triggered by situations or thoughts perceived as distressing. For instance, a survivor of sexual assault may avoid relationships or social outings out of fear of a recurrence. It's crucial to understand that this avoidance behavior has a purpose: individuals adopt it as a strategy to steer clear of threatening scenarios in an attempt to prevent a repeat of their traumatic experience (Tull et al., 2022).

The logic behind exposure therapy is grounded in the theory of classical conditioning (also known as Pavlovian conditioning), which describes the process by which humans and animals are trained to expect, and accordingly prepare for, certain outcomes (Gluck et al., 2020). Simply put, when one event (such as cloudy skies), often tends to precede a second event (such as rain), organisms learn to use the first event as a predictor for the second event. Therefore, if a person has learnt to associate cloudy skies with rain, they might carry an umbrella on days they see cloudy skies in order to prepare for the rain they expect to follow. According to Pavlov's model of classical conditioning, this association will only develop if the two events (such as clouds and rain) are paired together frequently. If the events stop occurring consecutively, a process called extinction occurs, and the organism stops expecting the second event to follow the first. In other words, if clouds appear often without rain following, then people stop expecting it to rain whenever they see clouds and will therefore stop carrying an umbrella on every cloudy day.

Some researchers believe that PTSD is associated with a decreased ability to extinguish such classically conditioned responses (Gluck et al., 2020). In this scenario, a person would continue to carry an umbrella every time they see clouds, despite the fact that clouds are no longer a good predictor of rain. In PTSD, these symptoms may present themselves through a person's continued emotional reaction to loud or sudden noises, despite the fact that such noises commonly occur without danger following. Exposure therapy aims to present such cues to patients within the safety of therapy so that the automatic, classically conditioned responses can be extinguished.

Using Pavlov's theory of classical conditioning, some researchers have found that a slight, but significant, adjustment to the way exposure therapy is currently conducted may elicit better results for PTSD patients. Normally, exposure therapy involves exposing patients to memories of trauma by presenting cues that trigger the memory, or by getting patients to recount the traumatic event. The idea is for patients to be trained to the extent that the cue no longer signals danger, by repeatedly exposing them to the cue without any negative consequences following (Gluck et al., 2020). A team of researchers in New York, however, found that instead of simply having nothing follow the cue, replacing a negative consequence with something new and neutral, such as a nonthreatening tone, leads to a better extinction of fear memories (Dunsmoor et al., 2019). To test their theory, Dunsmoor and colleagues trained healthy adults to expect an electric shock after seeing two faces (2019). Then, the participants were trained that the two angry faces would no longer predict a shock, which aimed to make the fear memories they had developed undergo extinction (Dunsmoor et al., 2019). Extinction was trained in two different ways. The first group underwent extinction using the methods that are typically used in exposure therapy, where the faces were presented and nothing happened afterward (Dunsmoor et al., 2019). The second group, however, were shown the two angry faces, and then were presented with a surprising, but neutral, tone instead of receiving a shock (Dunsmoor et al., 2019). This second technique has been termed "novelty-facilitated extinction," (NFE) (Dunsmoor et al., 2019). The NFE group showed much better extinction than the group undergoing classic exposure therapy, which indicates the novel stimulus, such as the neutral tone, facilitates extinction. The hope is that this knowledge can be applied to improve current exposure therapy techniques for patients with anxiety disorders such as PTSD (Dunsmoor et al., 2019). Dunsmoor and colleagues (2019) believe that the reason why novelty-facilitated extinction works better than typical exposure therapy is because it takes advantage of the brain's tendency to focus on new or unexpected stimuli. The novel tone presented after the cue is more memorable than the mere absence of a negative stimulus, which makes extinction more effective. Further research was done to find that people who had better prediction-related signaling throughout extinction learning displayed a better overall outcome with exposure therapy (Lange et al., 2020). Such findings alter the understanding and validity of certain exposure therapy processes, proving that these treatments are continuously evolving as scientists and doctors learn more.

PHARMACOLOGICAL TREATMENTS

This review highlights the potential effectiveness of trauma-focused psychotherapy (TFP) and pharmacological treatments in alleviating PTSD symptoms and improving patients" quality of life. It underscores the importance of rigorous research to determine optimal treatment components for TFP and explores promising avenues such as mindfulness-based interventions and virtual reality therapy. Well-designed trials are crucial to ensure the safety and efficacy of emerging therapies.

Additionally, personalized treatments based on biomarkers and genetic factors hold promise for enhancing treatment outcomes. While psychotherapy appears more effective than pharmacological interventions, there is a lack of research on medication efficacy for PTSD. Although some drugs may complement psychotherapy, their associated risks warrant caution. Despite current limitations, expanding knowledge about PTSD mechanisms and biomarkers may lead to more promising treatments in the future. Ultimately, bridging the gap between research and practice is essential for making evidence-based interventions accessible to those with PTSD. (Mansour et al., 2023.)

SUSCEPTIBILITY

Many people experience trauma in their lives, but only about 20% of those who experience trauma develop posttraumatic stress disorder (The Recovery Village, 2021). What makes some people more susceptible to PTSD? As with virtually all studies of susceptibility, the answer is a mixture of different factors. There is evidence that genetic factors play a role in a person's susceptibility to developing PTSD, as do social factors such as support from family and friends, prior life experiences, and personality traits (Gluck et al., 2020). PTSD is more common in women than in men, with approximately 8% of adult women affected compared to 4% of men, despite men experiencing more traumatic events overall. This gender difference may be influenced by the higher likelihood of women experiencing sexual assault and trauma (The Recovery Village, 2023). In many cases, environmental factors interact with genetic factors to determine a person's vulnerability to PTSD, so susceptibility can vary across a person's lifespan as their circumstances change (Alexander et al., 2020).

This comprehensive chapter explores the intricate relationship between trauma and the brain, shedding light on how traumatic experiences can precipitate posttraumatic stress disorder (PTSD) and influence various aspects of daily life. It delves into the intricate mechanisms by which trauma alters brain structure and function, particularly focusing on key regions like the amygdala, hippocampus, and prefrontal cortex (Lebow, 2021). The discussion elucidates how trauma-induced changes in these brain regions contribute to the development and perpetuation of PTSD symptoms. For example, the amygdala's heightened sensitivity to perceived threats can lead to persistent feelings of anxiety and hypervigilance, while alterations in the hippocampus may impair memory and exacerbate emotional reactivity. Additionally, the suppression of the prefrontal cortex, responsible for rational decision-making, can exacerbate fear responses and hinder emotional regulation. Moreover, the chapter examines the practical implications of these neurobiological changes on individuals' daily functioning. It delineates how symptoms such as rage, anxiety, flashbacks, and nightmares can significantly impact interpersonal relationships, work performance, and overall quality of life. Furthermore, it highlights the pervasive nature of trauma-related symptoms, including difficulties in concentration, learning, and decision-making, which can impede one's ability to navigate daily responsibilities effectively. In essence, this insightful exploration not only underscores the profound impact of trauma on brain functioning but also elucidates the complex interplay between neurobiology and psychological well-being. By comprehensively elucidating the neurological underpinnings of PTSD symptoms, this provides valuable insights into potential avenues for intervention and underscores the importance of trauma-informed care in supporting individuals affected by PTSD (Lebow, 2021).

Moreover, the chapter discusses the role of neuroplasticity in shaping the brain's response to trauma, highlighting the potential for adaptive changes and recovery. It underscores the importance of early intervention and evidence-based treatments in mitigating the long-term effects of trauma on brain function. Additionally, this research explores emerging research on novel therapeutic approaches, such as mindfulness-based interventions and neurofeedback training, in modulating brain activity and promoting resilience. Furthermore, it addresses the need for a multidisciplinary approach to trauma care, emphasizing the collaboration between mental health professionals, neuroscientists, and other healthcare providers. The research also delves into the impact of sociocultural factors, such as socioeconomic status and cultural beliefs, on the manifestation and treatment of trauma-related symptoms (Lebow, 2021). Furthermore, it highlights the importance of trauma-informed practices in various settings, including schools, workplaces, and healthcare facilities, to create safe and supportive environments for trauma survivors. Furthermore, the research explores the potential long-term consequences of untreated trauma on physical health, emphasizing the link between PTSD and chronic medical conditions such as cardiovascular disease and autoimmune disorders. Additionally, it discusses the role of social support networks and community resources in promoting resilience and facilitating recovery from trauma. Furthermore, the chapter addresses the need for ongoing research and advocacy efforts to raise awareness about the impact of trauma on brain health and to advocate for accessible and equitable mental health services for all individuals affected by trauma. In conclusion, this comprehensive exploration underscores the multifaceted nature of 'trauma's impact on the brain and underscores the importance of holistic approaches to trauma care that address both neurobiological and psychosocial factors (Lebow, 2021).

The cause of reduced hippocampal volume in PTSD remains uncertain, whether it's a consequence of developing the disorder, or due to genetic or biological predispositions. In studies involving identical twins discordant for trauma exposure and PTSD, the twin not exposed to trauma showed smaller hippocampal volume compared to twin pairs without PTSD, indicating that shared genetics and early environment increase vulnerability to stress-related disorders.

While some research suggests that trauma itself is linked to decreased hippocampal volume, other studies haven't confirmed this. Stress hormones, particularly glucocorticoids, may contribute to hippocampal volume reduction due to trauma, as the hippocampus is sensitive to these hormones. Our recent study found a negative association between childhood trauma and hippocampal volume, but this association became insignificant after adjusting for PTSD due to high collinearity between the two factors. Genetics may provide insights into causality, as gene variants precede trauma exposure and psychopathology (Zheng et al., 2021). Apart from the hippocampus, the amygdala, crucial for fear response and fear memory encoding, is frequently implicated in PTSD symptoms, particularly intrusive ones. Our consortium's study showed a nominal association between lower amygdala volume and PTSD and childhood trauma, though this "association's significance" didn't survive multiple-testing correction. Other brain structures involved in PTSD include the caudate, nucleus accumbens, and thalamus (Zheng et al., 2021).

Genetics significantly influences hippocampal structure, with high heritability observed in twin studies. Single genetic variants predicting hippocampal volume are well-established in nonclinical populations, and polygenic scores offer a simple method to assess genetic risk. These scores, derived from well-powered genome-wide association studies, explain more variance than individual risk variants (Zheng et al., 2021).

Our study aimed to use genetic variants associated with subcortical volumes to compute polygenic scores for the hippocampus, amygdala, and other structures in a target sample enriched for childhood trauma and PTSD. We hypothesized that environmental factors, particularly childhood trauma, would interact with genetic factors, as measured by polygenic scores, to predict hippocampal and amygdala volume. We also hypothesized similar interactions with PTSD diagnosis. We investigated gene-environment interactions using two approaches: modeling polygenic scores by environment interaction and conducting a gene-environment genome-wide association study in our sample. Due to limited data on adult trauma exposure, our hypotheses primarily focused on the hippocampus and amygdala (Zheng et al., 2021).

The studies mentioned previously are but a few that belong to a vast body of research exploring genetic and environmental factors pertaining to the risk of developing posttraumatic stress disorder. Future studies will build on those already available. Some may explore other factors such as personality traits. For instance, some studies have found that people higher in neuroticism, and those who tend to avoid novel situations, may have a higher risk of developing PTSD (Gluck et al., 2020). Others have found that those with a strong support system composed of family and friends have a lower chance of developing PTSD (Gluck et al., 2020). Some studies have even found that measures meant to prevent PTSD have led to increased rates of the disorder (Gluck et al., 2020); a phenomenon that will be important to further investigate to avoid inadvertently sending people down the wrong path.

CONCLUSION

In conclusion, with PTSD becoming increasingly salient in modern society, it is inevitable that research in this field will continue to grow. PTSD can be devastating if left untreated. Its significant interference with daily functioning can ruin relationships and throw a person's entire life off balance, which then causes ripple effects into wider society. With the field being so young, there is still so much to contribute to PTSD research, and many questions left to be answered. The more research that is conducted on PTSD, the more understanding people will have about the condition, which should lead to the development of more effective treatments and preventative measures.

One of the best ways to answer questions about the causal effects of trauma on the brain is to conduct neurological and psychological evaluations on people before they are exposed to trauma. While this may be challenging to do for the general population, it is an option that should be seriously considered for military personnel, many of whom develop PTSD after their service. The data collected prior to traumatic exposure can then be compared with data collected after exposure. These comparisons might yield insights that could be invaluable for understanding PTSD both in military veterans as well as in survivors of other types of traumas, such as asylum seekers, assault victims, and victims of natural disasters.

Overall, the better researchers understand the functions of the human brain, the better they can understand disorders such as PTSD, and the more likely it will be that fewer people will have to struggle with symptoms in the long term.

REFERENCES

Alexander, K. S., R. Nalloor, K. M. Bunting, and Vazdarjanova. "Investigating Individual Pre-trauma Susceptibility to a PTSD-Like Phenotype in Animals." Frontiers in Systems Neuroscience, January 14, 2020. https://www.ncbi.nlm.nih.gov/pmc/articles/PMC6971052/

American Psychological Association. "Cognitive Processing Therapy (CPT)." February 25, 2021. https://www.apa.org/ptsd-guideline/patients-and-families/cognitive-processing-therapy

———. "PTSD Treatments. Clinical Practice Guideline for the Treatment of Posttraumatic Stress Disorder." June 2020. https://www.apa.org/ptsd-guideline/treatments

"The Dangers of Untreated PTSD." Black Bear Lodge, n.d. https://blackbearrehab.com/mental-health/ptsd/the-dangers-of-untreated-ptsd/

Dunsmoor, J. E., M. C. W. Kroes, J. Li, N. D., Daw, H. B. Simpson, and E. A. Phelps. "Role of Human Ventromedial Prefrontal Cortex in Learning and Recall of Enhanced Extinction." *Journal of Neuroscience*, April 24, 2019. https://doi.org/10.1523/jneurosci.2713-18.2019.

Gluck, M. A., E. Mercado, and C. A. Meyers. "Learning and Memory (4th ed.). . Macmillan Learning for Instructors." 2020. https://www.macmillanlearning.com/college/us/product/Learning- and-Memory/p/1319107389

Lange, I., L. Goossens, S. Michielse, J. Bakker, B. Vervliet, M. Marcelis, M. Wichers, J. van Os, T. van Amelsvoort, and K. Schruers. "Neural Responses During Extinction Learning Predict Exposure Therapy Outcome in Phobia: Results from a Randomized-Controlled Trial." *Neuropsychopharmacology* 45, no. 3: 534–41, February 2020. https://doi.org/10.1038/s41386-019-0467-8

Lebow, H. I. "Can You Recover from Trauma?" Psych Central, June 3, 2021. https://psychcentral.com/health/trauma-therapy

Mansour M, Joseph GR, Joy GK, Khanal S, Dasireddy RR, Menon A, Barrie Mason I, Kataria J, Patel T, Modi S. "Post-traumatic Stress Disorder: A Narrative Review of Pharmacological and Psychotherapeutic Interventions." *Cureus* 15, no. 9: e44905, September 8, 2023. https://doi: 10.7759/cureus.44905

The Recovery Village. "PTSD Facts and Statistics." The Recovery Village. The Recovery Village Drug and Alcohol Rehab, April 22, 2021. https://www.therecoveryvillage. com/mental-health/ptsd/related/ptsd-statistics/#:~:text=Some%20interesting%20facts%20about%20PTSD,PTSD%20in%20a%20 given%20year

———. "Important Facts and Statistics About PTSD." The Recovery Village Drug and Alcohol Rehab. August 31, 2023. https://www.therecoveryvillage.com/mental-health/ptsd/ptsd-statistics/

Sloan D. M., B. P. Marx, P. A. Resick, S. Young-McCaughan, K. A. Dondanville, C. L. Straud, J. Mintz, B. T. Litz, and A. L. Peterson. "Effect of Written Exposure Therapy vs. Cognitive Processing Therapy on Increasing Treatment Efficiency Among Military Service Members with Posttraumatic Stress Disorder: A Randomized Noninferiority Trial." *JAMA Network Open* ;5, no. 1:e2140911, January 2022. https://doi: 10.1001/jamanetworkopen.2021.40911

Tull, M. "Exposure Therapy for Treating Post-Traumatic Stress Disorder Symptoms." Verywell Mind, January 22, 2022. https://www.verywellmind.com/exposure-therapy-for-ptsd-2797654

Zheng, Y., M. E. Garrett, D. Sun, et al. "Trauma and Posttraumatic Stress Disorder Modulate Polygenic Predictors of Hippocampal and Amygdala Volume." *Translational Psychiatry* 11: article 637, December 2021. https://doi.org/10.1038/s41398-021-01707-x

CHAPTER 15

THE GENERAL PUBLIC'S KNOWLEDGE ABOUT PTSD

There is an overall stigma associated with mental health which makes it incredibly challenging to have conversations about mental well-being and treatment. Just like everyone has physical health, all individuals have mental health as well. While physical health focuses on the body's physical well-being, mental health focuses on thoughts, feelings, and behaviors. Despite the connection and importance of both physical and mental health, there exists a great level of stigma around mental health and mental illness. There are a wide range of resources that have increased the public's knowledge about physical health and diseases, however, mental health literacy has been neglected. Health literacy, a term coined nearly two decades ago, is defined as education and access to information which increases an individual's ability to understand the importance and means of maintaining good overall health. In the area of physical health, health literacy resource examples include videos, articles, and conversations about maintaining a healthy lifestyle, prevention workshops about different types of health conditions, awareness campaigns about different conditions, smoking, and drinking, and educational workshops and training for first aid. People are able to gain access to these educational tools on the intervention as well as in libraries and other educational institutions.

While the general public acknowledges and appreciates information on physical health, mental health literacy was a term coined as an extension of health literacy (Sweileh, 2021). Unfortunately, it is not talked about much and does not gain enough attention and appreciation. The goal of mental health literacy is to provide knowledge about mental disorders in order to decrease stigma and increase treatment and prevention efficiency (Sweileh, 2021). There are several different components of mental health literacy for the general public: enough knowledge to recognize specific mental disorders based on the level and type of distress experienced by the patient, awareness about the various risk factors and causes associated with specific mental health concerns as well as mental disorders, education on the various treatment and prevention options available for people suffering from mental health problems, and knowledge on where to seek information regarding mental health related topics. Due to the lack of mental health awareness, the general public is unable to recognize certain disorders like depression, schizophrenia, and posttraumatic stress disorder. In a global research study that wanted to explore the general public's knowledge of mental health conditions there was a search for mental health documents that found a total of 945 with the earliest document originating from 1997. Of the discovered documents, Australia was found to have produced the most information about mental health disorders, followed by the United States (Sweileh, 2021). After research revealed that health literacy made positive impacts on health outcomes, researchers determined that developing mental health literacy would contribute to better care for people suffering from mental health conditions (Sweileh, 2021). While almost 50% of the US population suffers with mental health disorders of some sort, there is a high instance of people not seeking or receiving any kind of therapy for their conditions (Sweileh, 2021). The conclusion to be made is that a lack of mental health literacy exacerbates stigma against invisible disorders and causes feelings of fear or shame to interfere with people seeking treatment.

To encourage individuals to seek treatment and feel supported, it is important to understand the public's level of awareness about posttraumatic stress disorder. The types of attitudes people have about PTSD depend on various factors such as their race and culture, level of education and sociodemographic factors. A public study was conducted nationally in the United States which found that people who were younger, Caucasian and pursued high levels of education had a much more positive attitude toward people with PTSD and with mental health struggles in general (Tsai et al., 2018). It also suggests that white people have a better awareness of PTSD and are generally good at recognizing symptoms associated with PTSD. In 2016, a national survey was given to participants in the United States. Part of the survey asked participants to answer eight questions on a 4-point scale, which would determine their attitudes toward PTSD. For example, participants were asked to rate whether they think the government should invest more in PTSD research and whether people thought that individuals with PTSD tend to be dangerous. Furthermore, their general knowledge about PTSD was also assessed through questions related to PTSD symptoms and treatment. The results highlighted that a high majority of individuals, about 76%–94%, wanted the federal government to invest more money into the research, training and education surrounding PTSD. An overwhelming majority of individuals, about 30%, also believed that people with PTSD pose a threat to society and must not be given any sort of firearms. People had good overall knowledge about PTSD but sometimes, the experience with trauma and PTSD symptoms were overestimated. Furthermore, the demographics of the participants were studied in relation to their responses and one of the key things to note is that the level of education plays a huge role in the types of attitudes people have about PTSD. Participants who had received a higher level of education were more aware of PTSD and scored high on the survey pertaining to general knowledge about PTSD. They were educated about treatment options and were more concerned about the safety of individuals who were diagnosed with PTSD rather than being concerned about the effect people with PTSD will have on the general public. In other words, individuals who were highly educated did not consider people with PTSD to be a threat but instead worried about how vulnerable and threatened they may feel by others around them. This suggests that if a community would like to decrease the stigma associated with PTSD, it is important to invest in educational tools that will raise awareness and improve the mental health literacy surrounding PTSD and mental health, as well as mental illness in general (Tsai et al., 2018).

SOCIAL ATTITUDES TOWARD MEN AND WOMEN WITH PTSD

Social attitudes toward those who suffer from a certain disorder explains a lot about the stereotypes that exist in society in regard to mental illness. Studies on the general population have strongly suggested that there exists significant differences when it comes to experiencing trauma and PTSD in men and women. It is surprising to note that even though men have reported experiencing higher levels of stressors and traumatic events, women are twice as likely to be diagnosed with PTSD than men. Many studies have looked into this statistic and proposed that perhaps women have a lower threshold of managing emotions associated with trauma, or the types of traumas experienced by women are more violent than the ones experienced by men. While these differences may contribute to women being more likely to be diagnosed with PTSD. It is important to note that the general public's attitude toward men and women with PTSD also has a significant impact in determining which gender is more likely to develop PTSD (Olff and Langeland, 2022). Empirical studies of social psychology have confirmed the existence of gender-based stereotypes that are prevalent in our societies. These stereotypes are the reason why men are expected to be strong, assertive, and good at hiding emotions that may make them appear weak. Alternatively, women are expected to be shy, vulnerable, and soft, and it is considered normal for women to feel and outwardly express a wide range of emotions. Studies have also shown that people react in a negative manner when they see either gender violating gender norms or going against the commonly perceived gender stereotypes. In a study seeking to understand how gender and race are observed on social media, revealed that women have considerably more representation on social media than men, which is not so much due to the higher proportion of females online, but rather observed as a traditional social norm wherein men would not participate in public discussions of mental health (Utter et al., 2020). The study involved investigators analyzing over 215 photos available on a specific social media platform that used the hashtags #mentalhealth and #health to determine gender, race, and subjects featured within the photos (Utter et al., 2020). They used chi-squared analysis on data sets provided by each investigator in the study to compare frequencies of male, female, white, and nonwhite subjects within each hashtag category (Utter et al., 2020). All the investigators in this study recognized heavier female to male content, as well as heavier white to nonwhite subjects in the photos that were analyzed, which led to the conclusion that white women were most likely to publicly discuss health and mental health (Utter et al., 2020). The social tendency where it is expected that men conceal any sort of emotional displays and withhold healthcare treatment until the situation is absolutely dire is also associated with the female prevalence in both mental health diagnoses and public mental health discussions online (Utter et al., 2020). As such, it is revealed that the real-world stigmas against both men discussing health and against mental healthcare exist in cyberspace as well, creating yet another barrier against men seeking help or treatment for any such conditions (Utter et al., 2020). Ultimately, the study revealed that a disruption to the current representation in social media might function both to reduce stigma against mental health by showcasing mental health care as a global cause for every person of every age, race, and gender (Utter et al., 2020). Essentially, the more that humans talk and share information online, the more like people are to both understand and destigmatize mental health conditions including PTSD.

MYTHS ABOUT PTSD

There are some common myths about PTSD that are prevalent and accepted by some members of society. These myths make it difficult for individuals with PTSD to deal with the stigma surrounding their mental health concerns (The Recovery Village, 2021).

The first myth about PTSD is that only individuals who served in wars—military veterans—will be impacted by PTSD (The Recovery Village, 2021). While it is true that many military veterans are affected by PTSD, it is incorrect to assume that only those who have served in wars and in the military are affected by PTSD. Anyone who either goes through firsthand trauma or witnesses secondhand trauma can develop PTSD. Some traumatic experiences that an average human may encounter which can lead to PTSD includes domestic violence, passing away of a loved one, sexual assault, or a natural disaster. People who have experienced trauma since childhood, such as child abuse, or have lived experience with depression and anxiety or work in stressful environments are more likely to develop PTSD. While it is true that military veterans are exposed to a high level of stress and trauma, anyone from the general public can be impacted by PTSD (The Recovery Village, 2021).

The second common myth is that PTSD develops right after an individual experiences a traumatic event (The Recovery Village, 2021). This is incorrect as it can take several months or even years for an individual to develop PTSD due to a traumatic event that occurred earlier in their life. Usually, when an individual experiences a traumatic event, many symptoms of distress arise which can be attributed to PTSD. Although, this is not the case with each individual. Those who do not develop symptoms associated with PTSD right after a traumatic incident but do so later on in their life are said to have delayed onset PTSD. There are many explanations as to why symptoms would develop later in life. Some suggest that because traumatic events have a significant impact on thoughts and feelings, it may alter how memory is stored in the brain. Individuals who are experiencing ongoing trauma may suppress those thoughts and memories to cope but they may resurface back in their lives at a later point. Therefore, it is important to acknowledge that PTSD can impact people at a later stage in life and their feelings and struggles should still be validated (The Recovery Village, 2021).

Another incorrect assumption that people have about PTSD is that it is considered as a sign of weakness (The Recovery Village, 2021). It should be noted that this assumption, though highly prevalent in the general public, is absolutely incorrect. PTSD is a disorder that impacts an individual's cognitive abilities and how their brain perceives threats and deals with past trauma. Due to traumatic experiences, the victim's brain is wired to be on high alert and their fear response is heightened. The feelings and behaviors that emerge due to PTSD are not voluntary but rather extremely distressing for the individual. They are a form of coping mechanism that protects the victim from potential danger or threats and therefore must not be assorted as a sign of weakness (The Recovery Village, 2021).

A common yet incorrect idea that many people have about trauma is that anyone who experiences a traumatic event will develop PTSD (The Recovery Village, 2021). The truth is that not everyone who experiences trauma is diagnosed with PTSD. An American statistic states that while many people go through traumatic incidents, only about 6.8% of them develop PTSD. Whether or not an individual develops PTSD is linked to a few different factors such as sex, socioeconomic status, and previous mental health conditions. For example, women, people belonging to a low socioeconomic status, and those with previously diagnosed mental health conditions are more likely to develop PTSD after experiencing a traumatic incident. Other individuals who may have a high threshold for trauma, stress tolerance, and have various different types of support, may not necessarily develop PTSD following a traumatic event (The Recovery Village, 2021).

Another common idea that people have is that everyone with PTSD presents the same symptoms. This may be a common notion due to the media's depiction of PTSD and a generalization of what PTSD looks like, but this idea is incorrect (The Recovery Village, 2021). PTSD impacts people differently depending on the type of trauma experienced. People who experienced sexual assault may have PTSD but behave differently than a war veteran who has PTSD. Perhaps a sexual assault survivor does not like to be a part of large groups while the war veteran avoids loud sounds. The thoughts, feelings, and behaviors associated with PTSD are very different for every individual and should not be generalized (The Recovery Village, 2021).

A common myth about PTSD is that people who are diagnosed with PTSD have violent tendencies (The Recovery Village, 2021). This statement is incorrect, and it tends to increase the stigma associated with PTSD. Usually, people who experience PTSD symptoms tend to withdraw from their social environment or appear to be fearful and are always in motion in order to avoid any stressful situations. Only a very small number of individuals with PTSD appear to be violent. It is very likely that violence emerges as a form of self-defense from threat due to past trauma rather than a desire to be violent (The Recovery Village, 2021).

Overall, there are a lot of stigmas associated with mental health which makes it difficult to have meaningful and positive conversations. PTSD is one of the many psychological disorders that is portrayed in stereotyped ways in the media which has created various types of myths in the minds of the general public and as research has suggested, increasing educational material surrounding PTSD and mental health is important in order to decrease the stigma.

REFERENCES

Olff, M., and W. Langeland. "Why Men and Women May Respond Differently to Psychological Trauma." *Psychiatric Times*, April 27, 2022. https://www.psychiatrictimes.com/view/why-men-and-women-may-respond-differently-to-psychological-trauma

The Recovery Village. "8 Common Myths About PTSD." The Recovery Village. The Recovery Village Drug and Alcohol Rehab, April 8, 2021. https://www.therecoveryvillage.com/mental-health/ptsd/related/ptsd-myths/

Sweileh, W. M. "Global Research Activity on Mental Health Literacy." *Middle East Current Psychiatry* 28, no. 1, September 2, 2021. https://doi.org/10.1186/s43045-021-00125-5

Tsai, J., J. Shen, S. M. Southwick, S. Greenberg, A. Pluta, and R. H. Pietrzak. "Public Attitudes and Literacy about Posttraumatic Stress Disorder in U.S. Adults." *Journal of Anxiety Disorders* 55: 63–69, April 2018. https://doi.org/10.1016/j.janxdis.2018.02.002

Utter, K., E. Waineo, C. M. Bell, H. L. Quaal, and D. L. Levine. "Instagram as a Window to Societal Perspective on Mental Health, Gender, and Race: Observational Pilot Study." *JMIR Mental Health* 7, no. 10, October 27, 2020. https://doi.org/10.2196/19171

CHAPTER 16

HOW *PTSD* IS PORTRAYED IN MEDIA

Posttraumatic stress disorder (PTSD) is a mental illness that can affect anyone impacted by a traumatic event. While there is an increasing social awareness about the disorder, there remains a bulk of stereotypes and stigmas propagated and presented by the media. Nevertheless, it is critical to unpack these myths to better support individuals with PTSD. This chapter will discuss the depictions of PTSD in creative media like film, reporting media, and when applicable, social media. While PTSD can be experienced by any victim of trauma, this chapter will focus on the portrayal of war veterans and sexual assault victims with PTSD.

Despite both parties experiencing PTSD from traumatic events, there is a different tone toward combat versus noncombat trauma victims resulting in different stereotypes and hurdles. Veteran myths create the illusion of PTSD as a mental block that veterans can overcome through willpower since their soldier identities make them strong heroes, but ultimately, creative media depicts no treatment for PTSD. On one hand, the commemoration of war veterans and subsequent heroic portrayals are meant to be positive, but on the other hand, they are dismissive of veterans who return with scars that inhibit their reintegration into a society of productive members.

Moreover, victims of sexual assault suffer from victim-blaming narratives prominent in society and reflected in media, which combined with the lack of portrayal in reporting media relating PTSD to noncombat trauma, results in a massive hurdle toward seeking treatment. There are unique dimensions to the portrayal of PTSD victims depending on the circumstances and social biases. Not every dimension would be fully explored in this section but are nonetheless crucial to keep in mind.

Nonetheless, there are also commonalities shared by the two groups. The media portrayal of both groups reflects the lack of portrayal of treatment for PTSD, often focusing on the struggles with the symptoms, but no hope for treatment. Ultimately, the media must incorporate recommendations from mental health and PTSD advocacy groups to improve their portrayal of PTSD.

PORTRAYAL OF WAR VETERANS WITH PTSD

Generally, there is an increasingly accurate and sympathetic portrayal of war veterans with PTSD (Whitley and Saucier, 2022). In spite of this, there is a dominant discourse about veterans that is irrefutably intertwined with veteran myths. Whitley and Saucier (2022) analyzed representations of combat-related PTSD in popular Canadian news articles during a twelve-month period. Out of a total of 37,427 articles, 915 were usable for the study. Findings from studies such as these affirm that there is a limited understanding of PTSD, and that the postwar experiences of actual veterans' risks silencing veterans.

Whitley and Saucier (2022) noted that these articles most commonly depicted veterans in relation to themes of honor or commemoration for their services. Out of all veteran and PTSD-related articles, 53.8% discussed suicide and over 60% discussed some violent or criminal behaviors. These articles were often accompanied by stigmatizing language such as "ticking time-bomb" or "psycho." According to Whitley and Saucier (2022), this promotes the veteran myth of psycho-simplicity. Not only is this an inaccurate portrayal, but such media portrayals of PTSD are inaccurate and damaging by erasing true experiences and blaming victims of PTSD for not rehabilitating from their traumas and becoming productive in society.

Although the media in Canada has concerning portrayals, Whitley and Saucier (2022) also note that despite these negative connotations, over 50% of articles still portrayed veterans in a positive manner. Comparatively in the United States, the media portrays veterans less-so as victims and not with positive stories but instead focusing on trauma, emotional instability, and substance use (Whitley and Saucier, 2022). Vassar et al. (2020) agree that PTSD symptoms are commonly portrayed in war movies, but popular media perpetuates stereotypes, myths, and stigmas about PTSD by presenting a singular narrative. From studying fifty war movies, Vassar et al., (2020) found that 84% of the movies portrayed characters involved in US wars and developing PTSD symptoms. The authors discussed how one character, Michael from *The Deer Hunter*, reflected three main PTSD symptoms: hyperarousal, reliving the traumatic event, and avoidance/numbing. Vassar et al., (2020) saw that the most portrayed criterion for PTSD was exposure to trauma, standing at 59%, but avoidance symptoms were only shown in 9% of the movies. Whitley and Saucier (2022), however, found that the lasting image is of Michael overcoming his trauma because of his inherent soldier strength which allowed him to internally fight against his traumatic experiences in the same way he dealt with torture at the prisoner of war camp highlights the veteran myth of "unrecoverability." The individual would never be divorced from being a soldier. In addition, Whitley and Saucier (2022) found that war films continue to depict the myth of psycho-simplicity; the veterans all choose to ultimately "get over" PTSD. As well, Michael's rejoining of society remains within the conventions and norms, a continuous theme from the post-WWI and WWII films which expect victims of PTSD to act acceptably for society.

While news outlets in Canada portray a more nuanced depiction of veterans with PTSD than in the United States, they still propagate veteran myths (Whitley and Saucier, 2022). Canadian news is separated into two clusters of themes, with the first being Remembrance Day accounting for over 50% of articles. The second is murder, suicide, and sexual misconducts where the veteran's status as a veteran is brought up even if the article's main topic is unrelated to their service. Although PTSD and suicide are also comorbid with other mental illnesses, only 1.7% of articles discussed depression or anxiety. Although Whitley and Saucier's study was only a snapshot of articles in one year, Vassar et al.'s (2020) research affirms their findings. Over time from movies in the 1930s to modernity, PTSD symptoms have changed from being portrayals of various PTSD symptoms to narrowly focussing on negative affect and traumatic event recall. Indeed, Vassar et al., (2020) found that only one character was displayed seeking treatment for PTSD.

Although the depiction of PTSD as a complex issue is more accurate, it leaves a negative image of war veterans with PTSD.

Ultimately, the representations of combat-affected veterans are imbued with veteran myths that hide negative combat trauma symptoms in acceptable socio-cultural practices, repeatedly missing the depiction of healing and treatment. Not only is this an inaccurate portrayal, but it also appropriates the tragic outcomes of war as meanings for patriotism and heroism. The glorification of war veterans dismisses the trauma, especially PTSD symptoms that are not socially acceptable. Vassar et al. (2020) agreed; they found that popular American war movies present a distorted and inaccurate portrayal of PTSD, leading to the stigmatization of war veterans. This is especially detrimental to veterans who are re-entering the civilian lifestyle.

As well, Negri et al. (2022) noted that media can also impact the likelihood of developing PTSD and not affect perceptions of the illness. Using both extant research findings and a longitudinal survey of participants during the COVID-19 outbreak in 2020, the researchers identified differences in impacts between formal and informal news media. Formal media refers to news outlets, whereas informal media refers to social media platforms such as WhatsApp and Facebook. Through their findings, Negri et al. (2022) noted that intolerance for uncertainty was the greatest identifying risk factor that might result in PTSD development and this risk is further heightened by greater consumption of formal media than informal media. Although there are differences between sources, the findings that media can ultimately affect viewership's long-term mental health is congruent with existing research. The findings align with Whitley and Saucier's (2022) observations about veteran-related films where PTSD depictions are more about stress symptoms nowadays than in the past. Moreover, Negri et al. (2022) saw that PTSD was typically constructed as a military-specific disorder, emphasized by the military and heroic language used in legislative proposals about PTSD. This is also reflected in news article headlines, where 296 (34.0%) of the headlines included words like "battle," "war," "combat," "soldier(s)," "veteran(s)," or "military."

Negri et al. (2022) found there to be three main portrayals with negative implications. First, the populations who experience PTSD are not properly represented. Sexual assault victims are underrepresented, and military populations are overrepresented, which Negri et al. (2022) suggest could contribute to the misconception that combat exposure is a necessary criterion for PTSD, inhibiting noncombat exposed trauma survivors from seeking treatment. This is further exacerbated by the declining discussion of PTSD treatment in news articles. Second, many articles framed PTSD negatively, discussing court cases involving crimes, substance abuse, and presenting the negative stereotype of people with PTSD as dangerous or weak. This stereotype is a barrier to employment among military veterans, making reintegration into society more difficult. Third, Negri et al. (2022) found that most themes in the articles discuss causes and consequences of PTSD, but very few about prevention, risk and protective factors, and treatment. Without increasing the scope of PTSD to cover narratives about resiliency and recovery, instead of focusing on the social determinants of traumatic stress, PTSD is, like the movies post-9/11, presented in news media as a bleak disorder without hope. Negri et al. (2022) recognizes their limitations to one national US newspaper but asserts that the portrayal of PTSD in major news outlets needs to broaden in scope and ensure that they are not propagating negative myths and stereotypes.

PORTRAYAL OF SEXUAL ASSAULT VICTIMS WITH PTSD

Rape myths are common in media, and they irrefutably negatively impact victims of sexual assault. According to Vangeel et al. (2020), the two most common rape myths are that victims lie about rape when they regret consensual sex, and the victim is to be blamed for the rape because of either a provocative outfit or suggestive behavior. Rape myths are harmful in a variety of ways: they demoralize victims, support perpetrators, and shift the blame to the victims.

Rape myths make people believe that rape can be prevented by not becoming like rape victims, which denigrates the victims and lulls people into a false sense of security (Vangeel et al., 2020). In these ways, the media portrayal of sexual assault victims is largely unsympathetic, subsequently impacting the portrayal of sexual assault victims with PTSD. It is necessary to examine how sexual assault victims are depicted before focusing on the sexual assault victims with PTSD to situate within the larger context.

Borgogna et al. (2020) conducted a self-report survey study on relationship perceptions of men and women and the relationship of this with viewing pornography. In their study, the researchers described the "playboy" or "playgirl" norm, which is when an individual internalizes hypermasculinized, heterosexual discourse that ignores patriarchal roots of sexual violence against women and promotes ambiguous narratives that can both reinforce and propagate rape myths. Borgogna et al. (2020) found that as exposure to pornography increased, views, in particular men, were more likely to adhere to "playboy" or "playgirl" views and result in relationship problems. Indeed, research has shown that people who consume pornographic movies and magazines are more likely to accept rape myths (Vangeel et al., 2020). Vangeel et al. (2020) found that college women who watch more television are also more likely to believe that rape accusations are false. The data however did not indicate that television use correlated with more rape cases. Nevertheless, it is evident that creative media contributes to rape myths and misconceptions, placing more burden on victims of sexual assault.

Popular TV shows, specifically dramas, perpetuate misconceptions about sexual assault. While most sexual assault victims knew their perpetrator, this is not always accurately depicted in media portrayals of sexual assault in American fictional and nonfictional crime shows. Moreover, Ryalls (2021) conducted a study on representations of rape culture in recent teen television shows aired from 2016–2020 and found that although shows acknowledged the importance of affirmative consent, they continue to rely on the myth that that "no" may mean "yes." Shows such as *13 Reasons Why* and *Sweet/Vicious* may be helpful in emphasizing the importance of consent, but they also contribute to rape culture for this reason. The propagation of rape myths in media negatively impacts the social perception of rape, placing the blame on victims which can exacerbate trauma.

In the twenty-first century, social media is a key phenomenon in both reflecting and influencing perceptions of social issues. Andreasen (2020) sought to study how female victims of sexual violence were portrayed in Internet memes about #MeToo on the social media Web sites 9gag, Reddit, and Imgur found that the victims were divided into two categories: "rapeable" or "unrapeable" depending on their appearance and sexual agency. Like creative media, social media propagates rape myths centered on victim-blaming, but the presence on social media within a humorous discursive space provides another sinister element: it trivializes sexual violence. This study reveals several important elements: the backlash to a movement meant to provide a safe space for victims of sexual assault to come forward, the subsequent counter-movement, and the pervasiveness of rape myths across social media platforms.

The #MeToo movement began as a way for victims of sexual violence to share their experiences, revealing shared trauma and how sexual violence was normalized globally (Andreasen, 2020). Some mainstream media stories however framed the movement as a "witch hunt" against men and conflating "harmless" flirtation with rape (Santos et al., 2023). A movement about how, largely, women were abused by men became framed as a ploy to ruin the careers and lives of great men, a clear reflection of the rape myths in creative media. Andreasen (2020) references the notion of *himpathy* defined by Kate Manne as a significant and disproportioned sympathy given toward white men in regard to situations involving sexual assault crimes, domestic violence, murder, and other such traumatic crimes involving male-on-female abuse, which often results in the exoneration of the male perpetrator, shifting the blame to the victim. Clearly, the victim-blaming narrative is not prevalent in creative media, rather a social phenomenon amplified across all forms of media. Moreover, Andreasen (2020) noted that the 9gag, Reddit, and Imgur media websites were predominantly male-centric spaces, and so the portrayal of victims was mainly from a male-centric perspective.

Andreasen (2020) analyzed 866 Internet memes using the search terms #MeToo, Harvey Weinstein, Kevin Spacey, and Louis C.K, finding that child victims were portrayed significantly differently from adult female victims. Kevin Spacey was clearly highlighted as a pedophile and his search yielded very few memes about male victims, but this differed for the other searches. Of the 866 memes, 110 were about female victims, often discussing their sexual attractiveness. Evidently, this supports Santos et al.'s (2023) assertion that women's sexual attractiveness is often related to sexual violence, especially in virtual rape threats. As Andreasen (2020) adds, the credibility of women's accusations against powerful men is typically evaluated by the virtual peanut gallery by how they perceive the woman's physical attractiveness to determine if the man would find them sexually attractive. In this manner, sexual violence is reconceptualized as sex, both removing and trivializing the violence or force.

Contrary to the portrayal of war veterans, the traumatic event is often completely dismissed for female victims of sexual assault due to prevailing rape myths. Moreover, Masciantonio et al. (2021) found that Twitter users who produced victim-blaming content were more likely to be retweeted and have more followers than Twitter users who tweet victim support content. The research suggests that rape culture is, veritably, a core part of social media that must be further studied. Nonetheless, the perpetuation of rape myths, combined with a lack of news media relating PTSD with sexual assault victims, both silence and blame victims of sexual assault.

In conclusion, the cause for PTSD can be any traumatic event, but for this chapter, the focus was on the impacts of combat-related trauma and sexual assault. Despite the increasing social awareness about PTSD, many negative stereotypes and myths persist. In the depiction of war veterans, veteran myths continue to propagate ideas that dismiss the path of treatment. While creative media often accurately portrayed PTSD symptoms, they rarely, if ever, highlighted the healing journey. While there was a broad shift from wholly dismissing PTSD as a mental block to recognizing the complexities and difficulties of the disorder, there continues to be a lack of treatment depiction. As well, news media often portrays excessively negative stories without any empowering or constructive stories. Furthermore, news media overrepresents PTSD concerning war veterans and severely underrepresents PTSD experienced by victims of sexual assault.

Combined with the abundance of rape myths in creative media and social media, victims of sexual assault are, not only, often undermined, but also blamed for the trauma. While war is a recognizable trauma, rape myths and misconceptions can often reconstruct rape as sex instead of violence, further undermining victims of sexual assault. Indeed, there are dimensions to the portrayal of PTSD victims depending on social biases. While neither group is properly portrayed in media, the prevalence of misogyny, highlighted by the recent backlash to the #MeToo movement, adds another burden to female victims of sexual assault. This chapter is only a dip into looking at media portrayals of people with PTSD; there are many more dimensions to consider and explore in-depth to both properly support individuals with PTSD and dismantle harmful stereotypes, stigmas, and myths.

REFERENCES

Andreasen, M. B. "'Rapeable' and 'Unrapeable' Women: The Portrayal of Sexual Violence in Internet Memes About #MeToo." *Journal of Gender Studies* 30, no. 1: 102–113, 2020. https://doi: 10.1080/0 9589236.2020.1833185Borgogna, N. C., T. Smith, R. C. McDermott, and M. Whatley. "Are Playboy (and Girl) Norms Behind the Relationship Problems Associated with Pornography Viewing in Men and Women?" *Journal of Sex and Marital Therapy* 46, no. 5: 491–507, 2020. https://doi:10.1080/00926 23X.2020.1760980.4-8

Masciantonio, A., S. Schumann, and D. Bourguignon. "Sexual and Gender-Based Violence: To Tweet or Not to Tweet?" *Cyberpsychology* 15, no. 3: 1–17, 2021. https://doi:10.5817/ CP2021-3-4

Negri, O., D. Horesh, I. Gordon, and I. Hasson-Ohayon. "Searching for Certainty During a Pandemic: A Longitudinal Investigation of the Moderating Role of Media Consumption on the Development of Posttraumatic Stress Symptoms During COVID-19." *Journal of Nervous and Mental Disease* 210, no. 9: 672–679, 2022. https:// doi:10.1097/NMD.0000000000001518

Ryalls, E. D. "Representing Rape Culture on Teen Television." *Popular Communication* 19, no. 1: 1–13, January 2021. https://doi:10.1080 /15405702.2020.1868044

Santos, I. L. S., C. E. Pimentel, and T. E. Mariano. "Online Trolling: The Impact of Antisocial Online Content, Social Media Use, and Gender." *Psychological Reports* 126, no. 3: 1416–29, 2023. https:// doi:10.1177/00332941211055705

Vangeel, L., S. Eggermont, and L. Vandenbosch. "Does Adolescent Media Use Predict Sexual Stereotypes in Adolescence and Emerging Adulthood? Associations with Music Television and Online Pornography Exposure." *Archives of Sexual Behavior:*

The Official Publication of the International Academy of Sex Research 49, no. 4: 1147–61, 2020. https://pubmed.ncbi.nlm.nih.gov/32180100/

Vassar, M., A. Mazur, S. Hillier, R. Wilson, A. Demand, K. Lu, and D. Peyok. "Evaluation of Accuracy of Portrayals of Posttraumatic Stress Disorder in Popular War Movies." *Journal of Nervous & Mental Disease* 208, no. 7: 579–580, July 2020. https://journals.lww.com/jonmd/citation/2020/07000/evaluation_of_accuracy_of_portrayals_of.9.aspx

Whitley, R., and A. Saucier. "Media Coverage of Canadian Veterans, with a Focus on Post Traumatic Stress Disorder and Suicide." *BMC Psychiatry* 22, no. 1: article 339, December 1, 2022. https://bmcpsychiatry.biomedcentral.com/articles/10.1186/s12888-022-03954-8

17

PTSD AND THE *FAMILY*

Posttraumatic stress disorder can affect not only those who are diagnosed, but also those who are around the victim. Whether the relationship is close or a care-giving role, PTSD has the power to affect extensively. Living with a PTSD sufferer may become stressful for members of the household. There is likely to be heightened feelings of tension, anxiousness, depression, loneliness, confusion, and sometimes guilt. Consistent negative energy in the household can be emotionally burdensome. It is important to be aware of the different ways relationships can be affected and how to deal with the struggles during a patient's recovery.

WITHDRAWAL AND DISCONNECTION

Trauma survivors have difficulties maintaining intimate relationships. PTSD victims find it challenging to share their feelings with others and to make new connections interpersonally. Withdrawal and disconnection come hand in hand. There is great difficulty in articulating feelings and experiencing positive feelings. Having a strong line of communication between two people requires effort and maintenance. Many patients are unwilling to share their personal feelings and make social connections because they feel that there is little or no relation between their personal experiences, namely the trauma, and others' experiences. These emotional and behavioral changes strain the relationships the patient has with others when there isn't awareness (Villines, 2020). A way of seeing it could be that they are trying not to spread the negative feelings and experiences they have had. It's normal for PTSD victims to keep to themselves. This behavior, however, can lead to the loss of their support system and close relationships.

SYMPATHY

Family members and friends usually have sympathy for a PTSD victim when they are aware of the trauma that has occurred. Although showing sympathy is a way for family members to show their care, from the perspective of the trauma victim, it is not helpful. Rather than showing sympathy, close family and friends of the trauma victim should not treat or see them as a different person (Larsen, n.d.). Acknowledging the traumatic experience is the first step, but sympathy should not overstep the bounds of interaction. Interactions should remain relatively similar. Sympathy causes the victim to have negative feelings and they begin to feel that the trauma has caused the relationships they have with others to change in a way that they don't want. It produces insecurity and the opinion that the trauma has caused the PTSD victim to become a weaker person. This then spirals into low self-esteem and low self-expectations.

CONFLICT AND ANGER

A serious issue for many, if not most PTSD victims, is that they find themselves becoming more irritable with their family and those around them. Conflict is often a result of situations that do not go as planned or expected, the loss of control in their daily lives. Mistrust also contributes to their impatience and frustration. As mentioned before, withdrawal and the feeling that others cannot relate to their traumatic experience, causes the victims to frequently feel that they have been misunderstood or others are unable to understand (Villines, 2020). These negative feelings often lead to anger. With consistent conflict within a family, it can be difficult to manage due to increased tension and high tension within the family dynamic.

Anger is a contributing factor to conflict within families dealing with PTSD. Much of their distress can be due to the victim's inability to move on from the trauma or the perpetrator of the trauma. It is also possible for family members to be unaware that victims are not making a conscious choice in allowing the trauma to affect their lives in the way that it has socially and psychologically. It is an easy trap for friends and family of PTSD sufferers to return to irritable behavior with frustration and anger. A negative home environment can possibly lead to substance abuse.

GUILT

It is not uncommon for people to feel guilty and helpless toward a family member suffering from PTSD. Whether it be failure to prevent the trauma from happening or little improvement during the recovery process, there is a sense of responsibility and inability that is present. Particularly with cases of patients showing severe symptoms of depression and anxiety, these adverse feelings have an effect on the family dynamic. These feelings of guilt may lead to obvious and unwanted sympathy that does not support a positive recovery progression and process.

AVOIDANCE

Although avoidance and disconnection are behavioral symptoms of PTSD sufferers, family members engage in avoidance in another way. Trauma victims evade stimuli and social interactions, including trauma-related conversations (Tull, 2023). Family members and friends' frequent response to a PTSD victim's avoidance is also avoidance. As the victim is uncomfortable addressing the topic, people around the victim also tend to abstain from social reminders. Addressing the trauma in a clinical or therapeutic standpoint is important for recovery and moving on. Sweeping the issue aside does not contribute to the healing process. But uninformed confrontation may result in adverse feelings and anger from a PTSD sufferer.

DEPRESSION

The depression experienced by PTSD sufferers mainly stems from traumatic events. Trauma victims have feelings of uncertainty because trauma is unpredictable. An environment that was once considered to be safe can be changed into a place of doubt. What was once part of their everyday life is no longer the way the victim once knew it to be. It is difficult for victims to trust, and they often begin to doubt many other aspects of their life after being shaken by trauma, including family. In many cases, people with close ties to the victim need to earn and build trusting relationships again.

STRESSES FOR THE PRIMARY CAREGIVER

For most PTSD patients, there is one person that takes over the role as the main caregiver. When there is a significant other, this usually becomes their responsibility. The partner is challenged with the obligation of maintaining both their lives and duties within a household. This includes groceries, finances, and chores around the house. With the increase of tasks, the significant other serving as a caregiver can be overwhelmed and frustrated with their partner's inability to assume and share responsibilities. A caregiver can experience psychological stress and burnout that results in drugs and alcohol abuse, avoidance behavior, and negative emotions such as anger, depression, and guilt ("How to Treat Caregiver Burnout," 2023). As important as it is to care for a PTSD family member, it is equally important for caregivers to care for themselves.

Here are a few things in families affected by PTSD can do to take better care of themselves:

- Maintain a social life outside of caregiving duties.

- Join a support group, if there is none available, start your own.

- Create a family routine.

- Make time for every member of the family apart from the victim of PTSD.

- Take care of yourself and your health, both physically and mentally.

- If needed, seek professional assistance.

- Continue to learn about PTSD.

By better understanding how to interact with a PTSD sufferer, family and friends can effectively be a part of the recovery process. Reading books and doing proper research on the Internet with reliable sources can be invaluable.

At the end of this book there is a resource section as a starting point for research and where to seek assistance. There are online resources, books, worksheets, and a small directory of phone numbers and Web sites for North America, Europe, and India.

REFERENCES

"How to Treat Caregiver Burnout." Cleveland Clinic, August 16, 2023. https://my.clevelandclinic.org/health/diseases/9225-caregiver-burnout

Larsen, S. E. "Effects of PTSD on Family." U. S. Department of Veterans Affairs, n.d. https://www.ptsd.va.gov/professional/treat/specific/ptsd_family.asp

Tull, M. "Why People with PTSD Use Emotional Avoidance to Cope." Verywell Mind, November 16, 2023. https://www.verywellmind.com/ptsd-and-emotional-avoidance-2797640

Villines, Z. "PTSD and Relationships: Coping, Supporting a Partner, and More." *Medical News Today*, May 27, 2020. https://www.medicalnewstoday.com/articles/relationship-ptsd#ptsd-symptoms

18

RECOVERY AND HOW TO SUPPORT SOMEONE WITH PTSD

osttraumatic stress disorder, also well-known as PTSD, is a disorder in which an individual may develop mood, avoidance, or flashback symptoms after experiencing a traumatic or dangerous event (Mind, 2021). A temporary feeling of fear toward an experience is natural, but long-term symptoms may indicate PTSD. These symptoms may interfere with the individual's capability to work and maintain relationships (Mind, 2021). PTSD may occur in individuals who have experienced events such as dangerous accidents, deaths, injuries, sexual violence, and war (The American Psychiatric Association, 2020).

As of 2021, over eight million American adults live with PTSD, with 3.6% of the American population experiencing PTSD in the most recent year and 5% of the population experiencing PTSD at any time (Anxiety and Depression Association of America, 2021; Mind, 2021). In the Canadian population, 9% of individuals will experience PTSD in their life (McGrath et al., 2023). Canada is also one of the countries with the highest PTSD diagnoses (McGrath et al., 2023). Additionally, 20% of Americans who witnessed traumatic events also developed PTSD afterwards, and 11% of women are said to experience PTSD during their lifetime (Mind, 2021). With the prevalence of PTSD in society, it should be a priority to ensure proper treatment and recovery of diagnosed individuals. Many treatment types are available and have evidence to back up their functionality in PTSD recovery. Thus, this chapter aims to walk through an overview of the treatments and recovery of PTSD. Furthermore, it will explain how to help a loved one who is recovering from PTSD.

PTSD RECOVERY AND TREATMENTS

PTSD recovery is a complex matter and varies for individuals with different life circumstances and factors. Each and every experience is unique and different; some individuals may recover in a matter of months, while some may take longer (Mind, 2021). In addition, different treatments may work better for certain individuals while others may respond better to alternative methods.

Generally, recovery may be separated into stages (Pyramid Healthcare, 2020). Not all stages are necessarily experienced in recovery; however, progression through these stages may indicate recovery is occurring. First is the impact stage, also known as the emergency stage. This is the period of time directly after the trauma-causing event. This may be a stage of shock, worry, and guilt (Pyramid Healthcare, 2020). Next is the denial stage, where thoughts or feelings related to the event in question are attempted to be buried. This avoidance can manifest in different forms, such as purposefully or unconsciously refraining from painful emotions through, for example, alcohol use (Pyramid Healthcare, 2020). This however can also be the rescue stage, where the individual begins to understand and acknowledge the event that has occurred without the initial stressor emotions (Corrigan et al., 2020). Following that, a stage of short-term recovery may begin. An individual may try to gain normalcy in their everyday lives and try to address their PTSD with treatment or help (Pyramid Healthcare, 2020). They may, however, be plagued with problematic thoughts and fluctuating feelings based on the support they may receive (Pyramid Healthcare, 2020). Moving forward from that may be a stage of long-term recovery; this stage can help an individual deal with and overcome PTSD. Healing and treatment can help negate their symptoms and help an individual truly gain back a sense of order (Pyramid Healthcare, 2020). Treating PTSD can help prevent long-term symptoms and negative emotions made worse if it had gone untreated (Corrigan et al., 2020). Going through these stages may overall sum up the experience of recovering from PTSD.

What does treatment actually entail? Professional treatment of PTSD can include many different therapies and methods to help an individual move through the negative symptoms associated with PTSD. As an overview, treatment methods can be psychotherapy-based and pharmacotherapy-based; they may also include new technologies such as virtual reality (VR). Some may be more effective than others in certain situations, based upon factors such as perception and barriers to treatment. These will be further explained in the following paragraphs.

The first group of treatments, as previously mentioned, include psychotherapy-based treatments. Psychotherapy treatments rely on talking with a professional to resolve symptoms of mental disorders, such as PTSD (Mind, 2021). A prominent example is cognitive behavioral therapy (CBT) (Anxiety and Depression Association of America, 2021). CBT targets an individual's thoughts, behaviors, and emotions toward a certain problem (American Psychological Association, 2020b). It aims to take these thoughts and change them into more constructive or helpful ones in order to improve one's outlook on the situation. This can result in improved and more productive behavior. It is also an effective and widely recommended therapy for PTSD (American Psychological Association, 2020b). Other commonly used techniques within this sort of therapy are exposure therapy and cognitive restructuring (Anxiety and Depression Association of America, 2021). Exposure therapy involves helping individuals overcome their traumas by exposing them to their fears in a safe way. An individual is shown their fear through media such as writing, physical visitation, or visual images. This can help desensitize an individual to their fear and help them recover (Anxiety and Depression Association of America, 2021). In addition, cognitive restructuring is also another intervention used in CBT. Cognitive restructuring involves using facts and a realistic examination of an individual's trauma to better understand and shape a perspective on it. This helps to give a more level view and to avoid thoughts of guilt or incomplete memories (Anxiety and Depression Association of America, 2021). In total, this treatment helps to make a traumatic memory 'make sense' and assists the individual in stopping some of their negative emotions (Mind, 2021).

There are also specific methods of CBT that are particularly useful for treating PTSD. For example, there is cognitive processing therapy

(CPT) (Anxiety and Depression Association of America, 2021). This type of therapy is specifically aimed at traumatic events and its relation to how an individual may view their environment and their own self. CPT is determined to pinpoint an unbiased view on the cause and result of the trauma on an individual's mind. This may help individuals exit the loop of blaming or condemning themselves for the event and replace it with more constructive thoughts about the event instead (Anxiety and Depression Association of America, 2021). Generally, CPT will last twelve sessions. It is shown to be beneficial to victims of abuse, sexual assault, disastrous events, and war. (Schnurr et al., 2022; Stevens, 2020).

Generally, the process of CPT may proceed as understanding, processing, then modifying beliefs, at times through writing activities (U.S. Department of Veterans Affairs, 2020). First, psychoeducation on PTSD can help the individual notice automatic thoughts in their mind that may be fueling their PTSD, outlining their thoughts on themselves and the surrounding people and world (Stevens, 2020). Next, the therapist may attempt to alter any self-blaming or self-condemning thoughts, helping the individual confront traumatic thoughts and reprocess them in a different way. The skills learned during therapy can help an individual change their own outlook on the traumatic event, as the therapist may help them rethink their ideas on topics such as esteem, power, trust, safety, or more. Specifically, CPT is distinct from solely traditional CBT because it focuses on trauma, which suits PTSD patients (Stevens, 2020).

Another form of CBT is prolonged exposure (PE) therapy. PE utilizes strategies in behavioral therapy to help individuals overcome the challenge of facing traumatic memories (Anxiety and Depression Association of America, 2021). In long-term PTSD, confronting traumatic memories through a safe space in therapy aids recovery. PE will typically last eight to fifteen sessions, occurring on a weekly basis for approximately three months (American Psychological Association, 2020a). Similar to CPT, psychoeducation plays a part in introducing this therapy and teaching the patient about PTSD (American Psychological Association, 2020a). In the following sessions, PE then allows this confrontation through imaginative experiences such as discussions, or real-life scenarios in which people or situations can help facilitate the treatment (Anxiety and Depression Association of America, 2021). This is called imaginal exposure and in vivo exposure, respectively; imaginal would consist of a therapist guiding conversations on the experience, while in vivo would consist of out-of-office assignments to experience prescribed stimuli (American Psychological Association, 2020a). Through this, PE is another format that guides an individual to treating and overcoming PTSD.

Prolonged exposure is regarded as an effective, cornerstone, and first-line treatment for PTSD (Schrader et al., 2021). It was found that it is useful to reduce depression, anger, guilt, and other possible comorbid symptoms that may arise along with PTSD. As previously explored in this chapter, PE can consist of four main steps, which are psychoeducation, imaginal exposure, in vivo exposure, and the resulting emotional processing (Schrader et al., 2021). PE is also versatile and flexible as it is easy to disseminate and grasp by practitioners for use. Clinical data shows that it is tolerated the same amount as other treatments and encourages the reduction of symptoms in veterans continually throughout treatment. Clinical data also corroborates the general efficacy of PE for PTSD patients, including those with more complex cases (Schrader et al., 2021). For example, out of a study of ten military veterans, a consistent reduction in symptoms was shown in 90% of the sample, while 80% showed significant reduction in their PTSD condition (Schrader et al., 2021). Thus, the American Veterans Health Administration has also put in place a PE training program to better equip professionals to deliver PTSD recovery care (Schrader et al., 2021

Another addition to the types of CBT is stress inoculation training (SIT). This method is aimed to negate anxiety by equipping individuals with ways to cope and manage PTSD stressors (Anxiety and Depression Association of America, 2021). The particular skills trained in this type of CBT include breathing techniques and muscle exercises to encourage relaxation, among others. Thus, it is shown that CBT plays an important factor in aiding the recovery and treatment of PTSD.

Furthermore, other treatments for PTSD are also offered that are not included in the CBT umbrella. One of these treatment strategies is eye movement desensitization and reprocessing (EMDR). EMDR psychotherapy utilizes a repetitive movement or sound in addition to recalling the individual's traumatic memory (Anxiety and Depression Association of America, 2021). Thus, it is still a type of exposure therapy, but it adds the element of an eye movement or hearing stimuli (Anxiety and Depression Association of America, 2021). It makes the individual recall the traumatic experience while experiencing these repetitive stimuli (U.S. Department of Veterans Affairs, 2020). In doing so, EMDR speeds up the learning processes and lowers the emotions surfaced by the memory, aiding the individual in changing the way it is remembered. It is usually done once or twice weekly, for up to twelve sessions, and aims to help memories become processed, lowering the negative emotions associated with it (Stevens et al., 2020).

Furthermore, other therapies exist in PTSD treatment. For example, present centered therapy (PCT) does not focus on trauma, but rather focuses on educating an individual about trauma and coping strategies for stress instead (Anxiety and Depression Association of America, 2021). Narrative exposure therapy (NET) is another method that is more specifically used for patients with trauma related to community or socioeconomic experiences, such as refugees (Stevens et al., 2020). The therapist helps to contextualize an individual's life narrative, letting them understand their traumatic experience and delve into their identity. This allows them to better understand all their emotional and behavioral reactions to certain events in their life through exploring an autobiographical story (Stevens et al., 2020). Group therapy is another treatment for PTSD. It allows individuals to share their experience with people who have been through similar events, allowing them to collectively share their emotions in a nonjudgmental space (The American Psychiatric Association, 2020). Group therapies may also include family members, since they may be affected by a loved one's diagnosis (The American Psychiatric Association, 2020). New technologies, such as VR and computer-based therapies are also used to treat PTSD (Huang et al., 2022). For example, VR can allow for the simulation of a trauma-related experience; computer-based therapy can deliver easy-to-access, predetermined care (Huang et al., 2022). Thus, many types of psychotherapy and therapy types may be efficacious in treating PTSD in different scenarios and capacities.

In addition to psychotherapy, medication, like antidepressants, may be used to treat PTSD (Bajor et al., 2022). There are multiple types of antidepressants available for use. Selective serotonin reuptake inhibitors (SSRIs) are one type of antidepressants that can be used for PTSD treatment (Bajor et al., 2022). These drugs work as their name suggests—they inhibit the uptake of serotonin, which is said to help regulate anxiety and mood. SSRIs are well-researched and are found to be generally effective in treating PTSD symptoms (Bajor et al., 2022). There are, however, wide ranging dropout rates, even though it is usually better received than other antidepressants. Tricyclic antidepressants (TCAs) are another one of these antidepressant medications that were shown to be effective through various clinical trials (Bajor et al., 2022). Although, they may induce many side effects and can cause high dropout rates, even higher than SSRIs. Monoamine oxidase inhibitors (MAOIs) are another type of antidepressants that may act similarly to TCAs in terms of their mechanism; it, however, showed mixed results in trials, but had greater efficacy than TCAs. Despite this, it still shows high dropout rates (Bajor et al., 2022).

In addition to antidepressants, a medication named Prazosin has been used to control symptoms such as nightmares (Guo et al., 2022; Moore et al., 2021). Mood stabilizers like lithium, anticonvulsants, and benzodiazepines are also used; however, they each have their own niche (Bajor et al., 2022). Lithium can bring impacts on the CNS, but literature is limited. Anticonvulsants may help reduce symptoms and instability in emotions or responses. Benzodiazepines are a sedative that may need further research and care to make sure it is not abused (Bajor et al., 2022). Some studies may even claim that it is harmful (Moore et al., 2021). Other medication types can also be considered, but like most, would need careful consideration and research before prescription (Bajor et al., 2022; Moore et al., 2021).

Despite the bulk of treatment options in the forms of therapy or medication, the efficacies vary from individual to individual. CBT however is strongly recommended as a treatment for PTSD (American Psychological Association, 2020b). Psychological strategies are most commonly the first line of treatment for PTSD, found through a study on interventions for veterans (Moore et al., 2021). CPT and PE are highly recommended for veterans, where PE is shown to be 60% effective for this patient base. EMDR is also gaining traction after a past of mixed perceptions. As for pharmacotherapy, SSRIs are the first choice as there is evidence of positive impact from this medication (Moore et al., 2021). Other drugs may be considered based on patient response and effectiveness, although they are not as well substantiated by research. A combination of treatments can be used as well and can help target severe PTSD (Moore et al., 2021). Patient receptivity is also something that may be considered. For example, a study of women showed that they preferred PE over drug treatment if they were to have been diagnosed with PTSD; undergraduate students preferred certain treatments such as cognitive therapy and psychoeducation (Huang et al., 2022). All this empirical evidence suggests different treatments for PTSD can be considered when deciding a recovery and treatment plan for an individual.

HOW TO SUPPORT SOMEONE WITH PTSD

Working through a PTSD diagnosis may be difficult and daunting for an individual and their loved ones. Thus, it is important to provide support through these steps to recovery. The first step before recovery is receiving the diagnosis. As many individuals may wait years or even decades prior to seeking help, it is important to understand what barriers to treatment may restrict someone from receiving treatment (Moore et al., 2021). A study of war veterans found that barriers to treatment include inaccessibility to mental health services due to cost, location, and ease of enrollment. It then may narrow down to societal and cultural factors such as mental health norms in veterans or politics (Moore et al., 2021). Next, their environment plays a pivotal role, as loved ones, friends, or employers may influence the decision to seek treatment. Lastly, their own views are a large determinant of if a veteran seeks help; this may include intrinsic factors such as their own beliefs or perceived need to be treated, or extrinsic ones such as their insurance or knowledge on the subject matter (Moore et al., 2021). To help support someone with PTSD, one may aid them in overcoming barriers to treatment. For example, a study examined the expressed emotion (EE) of relatives of PTSD patients and their effect on PTSD treatment (Huang et al., 2022). Relatives who scored high on the EE scale, which represented a higher amount of hostility and negative comments in the patient-relative relationship, showed worse prognosis and results from treatment. This helps to demonstrate the correlation between social support and recovery in PTSD patients (Huang et al., 2022).

From this, how does someone support an individual recovering from PTSD? Some suggestions include educating oneself about PTSD to better understand a family member or friend (Mind, 2021). Another is accompanying the individual in various ways, which may include partaking in recreational activities, going to doctor appointments, exercising with the individual, and more (Mind, 2021). Listening can also play a large role in assisting a recovering individual. Other supportive behaviors include the willingness to share and provide a comfortable, unpressured, and understanding environment for the individual to share their thoughts and experiences. Be mindful to not dismiss or judge what they have been through and learn how to help them avoid any unexpected triggers (Mind, 2021). Proper communication, such as being a good listener and showing patience can be a major encouraging factor for recovery. In addition, family members or friends should ensure to make time for self-care and to set boundaries. This is because a healthy person can help foster better support for the individual with PTSD (Mind, 2021). As social relationships can affect an individual's journey through PTSD, it is important to be cognizant of this and support a recovering individual in any ways that are personally feasible.

In conclusion, PTSD is a complex disorder with many stages of recovery and types of treatment. Recovery varies per individual; psychotherapy and medication are just some ways that PTSD is treated, and while they make work for some individuals, they may fail for others. It is important to work with professional help to determine what is right for each individual. In addition, support for individuals with PTSD can help them better overcome this challenge. This may include helping them face barriers to treatment or socially supporting a loved one in a difficult time. Through increasing research and collective learning about PTSD, stigma can be reduced so that more individuals can be treated for this invisible wound.

REFERENCES

The American Psychiatric Association. "What Is Posttraumatic Stress Disorder?" The American Psychiatric Association, August 2020. https://www.psychiatry.org/patients-families/ptsd/what-is-ptsd

American Psychological Association. "Prolonged Exposure (PE)." Clinical Practice Guideline for the Treatment of Posttraumatic Stress Disorder, June 2020a. https://www.apa.org/ptsd-guideline/treatments/prolonged-exposure

———. "PTSD Treatments." Clinical Practice Guideline for the Treatment of Posttraumatic Stress Disorder, June 2020b. https://www.apa.org/ptsd-guideline/treatments

Anxiety and Depression Association of America. "PTSD Treatment & Facts." Anxiety and Depression Association of America, June 2021. https://adaa.org/understanding-anxiety/posttraumatic-stress-disorder-ptsd/treatment-facts

Bajor, L. A., C. Balsara, and D. N. Osser. "An Evidence-Based Approach to Psychopharmacology for Posttraumatic Stress Disorder (PTSD)—2022 Update." *Psychiatry Research* 317: 114840, 2022. https://doi.org/10.1016/j.psychres.2022.114840

Corrigan, J.-P., M. Fitzpatrick, D. Hanna, and K. F. W. Dyer. "Evaluating the Effectiveness of Phase-Oriented Treatment Models for PTSD—A Meta-Analysis." *Traumatology* 26, no. 4, 447–454, 2020. https://doi.org/10.1037/trm0000261

Huang, T., H. Li, S. Tan, S. Xie, O. Cheng, Y. Xiang, and X. Zhou. "The Efficacy and Acceptability of Exposure therapy for the Treatment of Post-Traumatic Stress Disorder in Children and Adolescents: A Systematic Review and Meta-Analysis." *BMC Psychiatry* 22, no. 259, 2022. https://doi.org/10.1186/s12888-022-03867-6

Guo, P., Y. Fang, M. Feng, X. Zhao, S. Wang, M. Qian, J. Huang, and H. Chen. "Case Report: Prazosin Augmentation for Treating Comorbid Treatment-Resistant Depression and Chronic Prost-Traumatic Stress Disorder." Frontiers Psychiatry 13, July 21, 2022. https://doi.org/10.3389/fpsyt.2022.803220

McGrath, J. J., A. Al-Hamzawi, J. Alonso, Y. Altwaijri, L. H. Andrade, et al. "Age of Onset and Cumulative Risk of Mental Disorders: A Cross-National Analysis of Population Surveys from 29 Countries." *The Lancet Psychiatry* 10, no. 9, P668–681, 2023. https://doi.org/10.1016/S2215-0366(23)00193-1

Moore, B. A., L. Pujol, and D. S. Shearer. "Management of Post-traumatic Stress Disorder in Veterans and Military Service Members: A Review of Pharmacologic and Psychotherapeutic Interventions Since 2016." *Military Mental Health* 23, no. 9, 2021. https://doi.org/10.1007/s11920-020-01220-w

Mind. "Helping Someone with PTSD." Mind, January 2021. https://mind.org.uk/information-support/types-of-mental-health-problems/post-traumatic-stress-disorder-ptsd-and-complex-ptsd/for-friends-and-family/

Pyramid Healthcare. "What Are the Stages of PTSD?" Pyramid Family Behavioral Healthcare, July 15, 2020. https://pyramidfbh. com/what-are-the-stages-of-ptsd/

Schnurr P. P., K. M. Chard, J. I. Ruzek, et al. "Comparison of Prolonged Exposure vs. Cognitive Processing Therapy for Treatment of Posttraumatic Stress Disorder Among US Veterans: A Randomized Clinical Trial." *JAMA Network Open* 5, no. 1: e2136921, January 19, 2022. doi:10.1001/jamanetworkopen.2021.36921

Schrader, C. "A Review of PTSD and Current Treatment Strategies." *Journal of the Missouri State Medical Association* 118, no. 6, 546–551, 2021. https://www.ncbi.nlm.nih.gov/pmc/articles/PMC8672952/

Stevens, N. R., M. L. Miller, and M. U. Shalowitz. "Exposure Therapy for PTSD During Pregnancy: A Feasibility, Acceptability, and Case Series Study of Narrative Exposure Therapy (NET)." *BMC Psychology* 8 no. 130, 2020. https://doi.org/10.1186/s40359-020-00503-4

CHAPTER 19

EPILOGUE

Let's think back to the introduction and the story of Samantha. Reread Samantha's story and what should come to mind is that her entire life was affected by what happened to her that night. She withdrew from her friends and family.

For individuals directly and indirectly affected by PTSD, it can appear as an impossible condition to survive. PTSD is beatable, victims need to know that they are not alone. People around them need to let the sufferer know that they have support around them, and encouragement is much needed. When social and psychological walls are built to reduce the chances of stimuli, the loss of support contributes to a sufferer's decline. Do not let PTSD victims feel that they are abandoned.

Due to negative stigma and feelings of shame, many trauma sufferers do not seek professional help. People who are a part of support systems need to encourage seeking professional help. It is extremely intimidating to seek help and speak to unfamiliar professionals about personal matters. There are many tests and questions that need to be answered by the individual prior to receiving proper care and diagnosis. Although these tests can be off-putting and uncomfortable, these tests are essential prior to treatment.

If a potential PTSD sufferer is unwilling to see a professional, it is important for them to have a positive attitude toward the situation and take steps toward a healthy lifestyle. By maintaining a healthy diet and staying physically active, the chances of the individual slipping into depression decreases. A lack of exercise and a diet of unhealthy food will increase risks of depression. A healthy lifestyle maintains natural endorphins in the body and gives the body energy without the side effect of mood swings. Learning breathing exercises and meditation can reduce anxiety and help with relaxation. It gives a sense of control over the mind.

No matter how severe the symptoms are of how affected someone, or your own, life has been affected by PTSD, the condition can improve and will improve when treatment is sought out and changes are made in the lifestyle. There is always something that can be done to work toward recovery. There are medical treatments, but also incremental efforts that can be made at home. It is equally important for the victim and their family and friends to have open communication and be honest about feelings. Communication helps people understand each other better and being more aware of one another will help ensure support is given. This also greatly reduces the chances of comorbidity, suicide, and substance abuse. Although a patient may not completely recover from PTSD, it is possible to live with and manage the symptoms. Staying informed on recent developments and research on PTSD so that you can support the victim well. You can survive PTSD only if you strive to survive it.

CHAPTER 20

PTSD RESOURCES IN NORTH AMERICA, EUROPE, AND INDIA

CANADA

This compilation serves as an initial resource for individuals coping with posttraumatic stress disorder (PTSD) across Canada's provinces and territories. While not exhaustive, it provides contact information, including phone numbers, addresses, and Web site details for accessible assistance. Notably, all listed resources offer their services free of charge.

Books

Presented here are five notable books addressing PTSD. These selections are particularly significant for their ability to explain PTSD in a straightforward manner, making the concept easily understandable. Written with both sufferers of PTSD and their support networks in mind, these books offer valuable insights into the daily experiences of individuals affected by PTSD.

The Post-Traumatic Stress Disorder Sourcebook by Glenn R. Schiraldi

The PTSD Workbook: Simple, Effective Techniques for Overcoming Traumatic Stress Symptoms by Mary Beth Williams

Trauma and Recovery: The Aftermath of Violence—from Domestic Abuse to Political Terror by Judith Hehrman

A Mind Frozen in Time: A PTSD Recovery Guide by Jeremy P. Crosby

The Post-Traumatic Stress Disorder Relationship: How to Support Your Partner and Keep Your Relationship Healthy by Diane England

Worksheets

This is a list of worksheets that can be used as a tool to assess an individual's understanding of PTSD. Included in this list are online resources that can be utilized as well as books.

Online Resources

http://www.mirecc.va.gov/docs/visn6/3_PTSD_CheckList_and_Scoring.pdf

http://media.psychologytools.org/Worksheets/English/Behavioural_Experiment.pdf

http://media.psychologytools.org/Worksheets/English/Guidelines_For_ Better_Sleep.pdf

http://media.psychologytools.org/Worksheets/English/PTSD_Formulation_ Ehlers.pdf

http://www.getselfhelp.co.uk/docs/STOPPworksheet.pdf

http://www.getselfhelp.co.uk/docs/PTSDThoughtRecordSheet.pdf

http://www.getselfhelp.co.uk/docs/PTSDmetaphor.pdf

Workbooks

The PTSD Workbook: Simple, Effective Techniques for Overcoming Traumatic Stress Symptoms by Mary Beth Willams and Soili Poijula

I Can't Get Over It: A Handbook for Trauma Survivors by Aphrodite Matsakis

The Way of the Journal: A Journal Therapy Workbook for Healing by Kathleen Adams

Post-Traumatic Stress Disorder Relationship: How to Support Your Partner and Keep Your Relationship Healthy by Diane England

Conquering Post-Traumatic Stress Disorder: The Newest Techniques for Overcoming Symptoms, Regaining Hope, and Getting Your Life Back by Victoria Lemle Beckner and John B. Arden

Life After Trauma: A Workbook for Healing by Dena Rosenbloom and Mary Beth Williams

The Dissociative Identity Disorder Sourcebook by Deborah Haddock

Directory of Resources

This is a small directory of both online and in-person resources that can be utilized in each of the provinces and territories in Canada. It offers a start for individuals who are seeking professional assistance.

British Columbia

AnxietyBC: psychological treatments for PTSD

Phone: 1 (604) 525-7566

Address: 101-631 Columbia St., New Westminster, BC, V3M 1A7

Web site: http://www.anxietybc.com

British Columbia Psychological Association: lists of psychologists

Phone: 1 (800) 730-0522

Address: 402-1177 West Broadway, Vancouver, BC, V6H 1G3

Web site: http://www.psychologists.bc.ca

Maven Health and Wellness: treatment for anxiety disorders

Phone: 1 (877) 313-8309

Address: 400–601 West Broadway, Vancouver, BC, V5Z 4C2

Web site: http://www.mavenhealth.com

Police Victim Services of British Columbia: victim services

Phone: 1 (877) 869-0720

Address: 120–12414–82 Ave, Surrey, BC

Web site: http://www.policevictimservices.bc.ca

Ending Violence Association of British Columbia: resources for community services and helping sexual assault victims

Phone: 1 (604) 633-2506

Address: 1404-510 West Hastings St., Vancouver, BC, V6B 1L8

Web site: www.endingviolence.org/about/programs_we_serve

Alberta

Psychologists' Association of Alberta: list of psychologists

Phone: 1 (780) 424-0294 or 1 (888) 424-0297

Address: Unit 103, 1207–91 Street, Edmonton, Alberta, T6X 1E9

Web site: http://www.psychologistsassociation.ab.ca

Maven Health and Wellness: treatment for anxiety disorders

Phone: 1 (403) 313-8309

Address: Suite 700, One Executive Place 1816 Crowchild Trail NW, Calgary, Alberta, T2M 3YZ

Web site: http://www.mavenhealth.com

Saskatchewan

Government of Saskatchewan: mental health services listed by region

Web site: http://www.health.gov.sk.ca/mental-health-contacts-post-trauma

Saskatoon Sexual Assault and Information Centre, services for victims of sexual assault

Phone: 1 (306) 244-2294

Address: 201-506 25 St., East Saskatoon, Saskatchewan S7K 4A7

Web site: www.saskatoonsexualassaultcentre.com

Manitoba

The Anxiety Disorders Association of Manitoba (ADAM): cognitive behavioral therapy for anxiety disorders

Phone: 1 (204) 925-0600 or 1 (800) 805-8885

Address: 100–4 Fort Street, Winnipeg, Manitoba R3C 1C4

Web site: http://www.adam.mb.ca

Manitoba Psychological Society: list of psychologists by expertise

Web site: http://mps.ca/referraltmp.aspx

Ontario

MacAnxiety Research Centre at the McMaster University Medical Centre, Hamilton Health Sciences, treatment for anxiety disorders

Phone: 1 (905) 921-7644

Address: 1057 Main Street West, LO2, Hamilton, Ontario, L8S 1B7

Web site: http://www.macanxiety.com

The Psychological Trauma Clinic at Mount Sinaï Hospital

Phone: 1 (416) 586-4800 ext. 4568

Address: 600 University Ave, 9th floor, Toronto, Ontario, M5G 1X5

Web site: http://www.mountsinai.on.ca/care/psych/patient-programs/trauma-clinic

Quebec

Ordre des psychologues du Québec, list of psychologists by region

Phone: 1 (514) 738-1881 or 1 (800) 363-2644

Address: Suite 510, 1100 Beaumont Ave, Mont-Royal, Quebec H3P 3H5

Web site: http://www.ordrepsy.qc.ca/en/psychologue/index.sn

Trauma Studies Centre (TSC), cognitive behavioral therapy

   Phone: 1 (514) 251-4000, ext. 3734

   Address: 7331, rue Hochelaga, Montréal (Québec) H1N 3V2

   Web site: https://trauma.criusmm.net/en/

Clinique des Troubles Anxieux de l'Hôpital Sacré-Cœur (Bois-de-Boulogne), psychological assessment of PTSD

   Phone: 1 (514) 338-2222

   Address: 5400, boul. Gouin West, Montreal, Quebec, H4J 1C5

   Web site: http://www.hscm.ca

Clinique pour Victimes d'Agression Sexuelle de l'Hôpital Hôtel-Dieu (CVAS), PTSD assessment

   Phone: 1 (514) 890-8000

   Address: 3840 St. Urbain St., Montreal, Quebec, H2X 1T8

   Web site: http://www.chumontreal.qc.ca/

Nova Scotia

Association of Psychologists of Nova Scotia (APNS): list of psychologists

   Phone: 1 (902) 422-9183

   Address: Suite 435, 5991 Spring Garden Road Halifax, Nova Scotia, B3H 1Y6

   Web site: http://www.apns.ca

Halifax Regional Municipality, victim services

   Phone: 1 (902) 490-5300

   Address: 1975 Gottingen S., Halifax, Nova Scotia B3J 2H1

   Web site: http://www.halifax.ca/Police/Programs/victimservices.html

Prince Edward Island

Dianna Cudmore Program Secretary: victim services

   Phone: 1 (902) 368-4582

   Address: 51 Water St., Second Floor, Charlottetown, PEI, C1A 1A3

New Brunswick

Mental Health Services

Phone: 1 (506) 847-6300 or 1 (506) 848-6623

Web site: https://www2.gnb.ca/content/gnb/en/departments/health/mental_health_services.html

Newfoundland

The Association of Psychologists in Newfoundland Labrador (APNL), list of psychologists

Phone: 1 (709) 739-5405

Address: LeMarchant Road, St. John's, NL A1E 0A5

Web site: www.nlpsych.ca

Sexual Abuse Community Services, services for victims of sexual abuse

Phone: 1 (709) 643-8740

Address: 127 Montana Drive, Stephenville, NL, A2N 2T4

Mental Health Crisis Centre

Phone: 1 (888) 737-4668

Victims Services for Newfoundland

Phone: 1 (709) 729-0900

Address: 315 Duckworth St., P.O. Box 8700, St. John's, NL

Yukon

Mental Health Services: clinic for mental health patients

Phone: 1 (867) 667-8346

Address: 4 Hospital Rd., Whitehorse Phone: 1-800-661-0408, local 8346

Web site: http://www.hss.gov.yk.ca/programs/health/mental_health

Victim Services and Conjugal Violence Prevention Unit: victim services

Phone: 1 (867) 667-8500 or 1 (800) 661-0408, local 8500

Address: 301 Jarvis St., Whitehorse, Yukon, Y1A 2C6

Dawson City Victim Services

Phone: 1 (867) 993-5831

Northwest Territories

Mental Health Clinic, treatment for those referred by general practitioners

Phone: 1 (867) 873-7042

Address: 4916 47 St., Yellowknife, NT, X1A 1L8

Nunavut

The Nunavut Department of Health and Social Services

Web site: http://www.health.gov.nu.ca/en/Home.aspx

Department of Justice, victim services

Phone: (867) 975-6170

Address: Bag 1000 STN 500, Iqaluit, Nunavut, X0A 0H0

UNITED STATES

This serves as a valuable introductory guide for individuals grappling with posttraumatic stress disorder (PTSD) across different states throughout the United States. While it does not encompass an exhaustive compilation, it furnishes a range of resources for seeking support.

Web Sites

Following is a varied and comprehensive selection of Web sites covering topics related to trauma and posttraumatic stress disorder (PTSD).

Substance Abuse and Mental Health Services Administration: 2022 National Directory of Mental Health Treatment Facilities

Comprehensive directory of drug abuse and mental health facilities in each city in every state of the United States.

Web site: https://www.samhsa.gov/data/sites/default/files/reports/rpt35992/MH%20facilities/MH%20Directory/National_Directory_MH_facilities_final_04272022.pdf

National Center for PTSD

Resource contains information regarding understanding PTSD, its types, assessment, prevalence, related problems, awareness, treatment, places to get help, resources for families and friends affected, for providers, apps, videos, scientific articles, clinical trials database, publications, health links and more.

Web site: https://www.ptsd.va.gov/

Proquest: PTSDpubs

Open access to scientific journal database containing articles on PTSD.

Web site: https://www.proquest.com/ptsdpubs/index

Anxiety & Depression Association of America

Web site on understanding PTSD, its symptoms, and statistics; includes resources at the end of the page.

Web site: https://adaa.org/understanding-anxiety/posttraumatic-stress-disorder-ptsd

PTSD and Addictions

People who have PTSD often self-medicate, which can lead to addictions. This Web site addresses PTSD and addictions.

Website:https://www.addictioncenter.com/addiction/post-traumatic-stress-disorder/

Real Warriors (U.S. Department of Defense)

Web site for veterans and their families; covers a range of topics, including mental health.

Web site: https://www.health.mil/Military-Health-Topics/Mental-Health

Gift from Within

A detailed and informational page on PTSD and its treatment.

Web site: https://www.giftfromwithin.org/

Traumatic Stress Institute

Organization dedicated to training organizations on trauma care through delivery of consultations, professional coaching, and research.

Web site: https://www.traumaticstressinstitute.org/

BetterHelp

Therapy Web site providing information on PTSD, its symptoms, and finding a trauma therapist.

Web site: https://www.betterhelp.com/advice/ptsd/

Wounded Warrior Project

Description of PTSD, combat stress, and traumatic brain injury (TBI); PTSD causes, symptoms, treatment, and resources for Veterans specifically.

Web site: https://www.woundedwarriorproject.org/programs/mental-wellness/veteran-ptsd-treatment-support-resources

National Institute of Mental Health

Description of PTSD, who gets it, symptoms, risk factors, treatment, how to help someone else, free brochures, sharable resources, multimedia, and more.

Web site: https://www.nimh.nih.gov/health/topics/post-traumatic-stress-disorder-ptsd

Medline Plus

Comprehensive information on PTSD and its different aspects.

Web site: https://medlineplus.gov/posttraumaticstressdisorder.html

US Department of Veteran Affairs: National PTSD Brain Bank

Human tissue bank that collects, processes, stores, and gives out research specimens for future scientific studies on PTSD.

Web site: https://www.research.va.gov/programs/tissue_banking/PTSD/default.cfm

American Psychological Association

Leading scientific and professional organization representing psychology in the United States.

Web site: https://www.apa.org/

United Way

Details which states in the United States have the best and worst access to mental health services.

Website:https://unitedwaynca.org/blog/mental-healthcare-access-by-state/

App

PTSD Coach App

Developed by the National Center for PTSD for Veterans experiencing PTSD symptoms.

Web site: https://mobile.va.gov/app/ptsd-coach

Books

Provided in this section are valuable resources in the form of books addressing the themes of trauma, post-traumatic stress disorder (PTSD), and the journey toward healing.

The Body Keeps the Score: Brain, Mind, and Body in the Healing of Trauma by Bessel van der Kolk

The Complex PTSD Workbook by Dr. Arielle Schwartz

The Post-Traumatic Growth Guidebook by Dr. Arielle Schwartz

Behavioral Activation for PTSD by Lisa Campbell

The Body Remembers: The Psychophysiology of Trauma and Trauma Treatment by Babette Rothschild

Complex PTSD: From Surviving to Thriving: A Guide and Map for Recovering from Childhood Trauma by Pete Walker

What My Bones Know: A Memoir of Healing from Complex Trauma by Stephanie Foo

What Happened to You? Conversations on Trauma, Resilience, and Healing by Dr. Bruce D. Perry and Oprah Winfrey

Trauma and Expressive Arts Therapy: Brain, Body, and Imagination in the Healing Process by Cathy A. Malchiodi, PhD.

Healing Trauma: A Pioneering Program for Restoring the Wisdom of Your Body by Peter A. Levine, PhD.

Helplines

988 Suicide & Crisis Helpline: 24/7, free and confidential support for people in distress, prevention and crisis resources for you or your loved ones. Includes chat/text, and ASL interpreter.

Phone: 988

Web site: https://988lifeline.org/

National Suicide and Crisis Lifeline (options for deaf and hard of hearing)

For TTY Users: Use your preferred relay service or dial 711 then 988

Website:https://988lifeline.org/help-yourself/for-deaf-hard-of-hearing/

Childhelp National Child Abuse Hotline

Phone: (800) 422-4453

Web site: https://childhelphotline.org/

Crisis Text Line

SMS: Text HOME to 741741

Web site: https://www.crisistextline.org/

National Domestic Violence Hotline

Phone: (800) 799-7233

Web site: https://www.thehotline.org/

National Sexual Assault Hotline

Phone: (800) 656-4673

Web site: https://www.rainn.org/

Substance Abuse and Mental Health Services Administration National Helpline

Phone: (800) 662-4357

Web site: https://www.samhsa.gov/find-help/national-helpline

Veterans Crisis Line

Phone: 988, then PRESS 1, Text 838255

Web site: https://www.veteranscrisisline.net/

Videos

What Is PTSD? (Whiteboard Video). Veterans Health Administration

Link: https://youtu.be/YMC2jt_QVEE?si=USpidLK7xggCnmrF

The psychology of post-traumatic stress disorder—Joelle Rabow Maletis

Link: https://youtu.be/b_n9qegR7C4?si=fbnTNlZuzAlj14NL

The Truth About Complex PTSD and Essential Recovery Tools

Link: https://youtu.be/WY05GnsNWQM?si=EtK3C_O1-W8YCwrx

Posttraumatic stress disorder (PTSD): causes, symptoms, treatment, and pathology

Link: https://youtu.be/hzSx4rMyVjI?si=WmK1TLTlbBi-0uDx

Trauma versus PTSD (Post Traumatic Stress Disorder)

Link:https://youtube.com/shorts/hJ5T27pKmhs?si=qu7PMXzcxnOHrSOc

EUROPE

These resources serve as a foundational reference for individuals in search of professional assistance in managing PTSD. This guide provides an overview of available support services.

Sweden

Below is a diverse and extensive collection of Web sites encompassing subjects concerning trauma and posttraumatic stress disorder (PTSD).

Living with PTSD

An overview of what PTSD is and its symptoms.

Web site: https://blog.swedish.org/swedish-blog/living-with-ptsd

Swedish Society for Traumatic Stress Studies

The Swedish Association for Traumatic Stress, or SSTSS, seeks to disseminate and expand understanding of psychological traumas.

Web site: https://sstss-org.translate.goog/?_x_tr_sl=sv&_x_tr_tl= en&_x_tr_hl=en&_x_tr_pto=sc

Denmark

The Danish Center of Psychotraumatology

In terms of study, treatment, and prevention of trauma-related disorders, the Danish Centre of Psychotraumatology is the country's leading institution.

Web site: https://www.sdu.dk/en/forskning/videnscenter_for_ psykotraumatologi

Dansk Rehabilitering

Dansk Rehabilitering is a specialized rehabilitation service that helps persons with PTSD, burnout, anxiety, and depression. It is available to veterans, law enforcement, prison staff, and emergency services workers.

Web site: https://danskrehabilitering.dk/home/

Norway

The Norwegian Centre for Violence and Traumatic Stress Studies (NKVTS)

Violence and traumatic stress are the subjects of research conducted at the Norwegian Centre for Violence and Traumatic Stress Studies (NKVTS). The mission of NKVTS is to support victims of trauma and violence. The center is globally focused and advances academic knowledge on a global scale.

Web site: https://www.nkvts.no/english/about-nkvts/#:~:text=The%
20Norwegian%20Centre%20for%20Violence%20and%20
Traumatic%20Stress%20Studies%20(NKVTS,on%20an%20
international%2C%20academic%20level

RVTS Sør

RVTS Sør is an information hub for psychological traumas. Their
diverse expert workforce uses programs, courses, and information
work to put knowledge into practice.

Web site: https://rvtssor-no.translate.goog/?_x_tr_sl=no&_x_tr_tl=
en&_x_tr_hl=en&_x_tr_pto=sc

Finland

Traumaterapiakeskus

To professionals working in various contexts with individuals suffering from trauma, they provide training, supervision, and consulting.
Additionally, they offer EMDR therapy in addition to individual,
family, and group psychotherapy.

Web site: https://traumaterapiakeskus.com/?lang=en

Psykotraumatologian Keskus

The Centre for Psychotraumatology is an outpatient mental health
facility. For adults, children, and families severely traumatized by
conflict, displacement, and torture, as well as those with refugee ori-
gins, our multidisciplinary teams offer assessment, treatment, and
rehabilitation.

Web site: https://www-hdl-fi.translate.goog/psykotraumatologian-
keskus/?_x_tr_sl=fi&_x_tr_tl=en&_x_tr_hl=en&_x_tr_pto=sc

Iceland

(Geðhjálp) The Icelandic Mental Health Alliance

In Iceland, families and individuals can receive mental health treatments via the Icelandic Mental Health Alliance. They provide
assistance to people coping with addiction and other mental health
concerns, in addition to counselling and therapy services.

Web site: https://gedhjalp.is/english/

Lithuania

Lithuanian Society for Traumatic Stress

> A summary of what PTSD is, its symptoms, and the details of using techniques such as EMDR and BEPP to work with patients suffering from trauma.

> Web site: https://traumupsichologija.lt/en/posttraumaticstress/#:~: text=In%20Lithuania%2C%20there%20are%20currently, Psychotherapy%20for%20PTSD%20(BEPP)

Pagalbos Linijos

> List of contact information for psychological support.

> Web site: https://pagalbasau.lt/pagalbos-linijos/

Estonia

Estonian Refugee Council

> In order to improve the psychological well-being of refugees and guarantee a healthier and more balanced society overall, their program provides a range of mental health-promoting activities, such as group and individual therapy sessions.

> Web site: https://www.pagulasabi.ee/en/programmid/mental-health-programme

Tartu Ülikooli Kliinikumi Psühhiaatriakliinik (Tartu University Hospital)

> An Estonian public hospital offering mental health treatments. They have a group of skilled psychologists and psychiatrists that handle medications for mental health conditions in addition to offering individual and group treatment.

> Web site: https://www.kliinikum.ee/patsiendile/erakorraline-vastuvott/psuhhiaatriakliinik/

Latvia

Find a Helpline

> Lists some Latvian mental and behavioral health support help lines.

> Web site: https://findahelpline.com/countries/lv

Karyn Purvis Institute of Child Development

Includes a book project that focuses on a how to deal with a child that has gone through trauma.

Web site: https://child.tcu.edu/the-connected-child-in-latvian/# sthash.oHWTo9jU.dpbs

Greenland

Psychology Today

Includes a list of therapists specializing in dealing with people who suffer from PTSD in Greenland.

Web site: https://www.psychologytoday.com/us/therapists/nh/ greenland?category=trauma-and-ptsd

Ireland

Centric Mental Health

An overview of PTSD, its symptoms, different types of treatments that can be used, list of different clinics offering treatments for it in Ireland.

Web site: https://mentalhealth.ie/post-traumatic-stress-disorder

PTSD—Anxiety Ireland

A clinic offering services for people suffering from PTSD.

Web site: https://www.anxietyireland.ie/ptsd/

United Kingdom

PTSD UK

An overview of the resources available to help with PTSD in the UK.

Web site: https://www.ptsduk.org/

UK Trauma Council

Resources to assist people and organizations that foster and safeguard children and adolescents who have experienced trauma. Created by top UK experts on childhood trauma, one may access articles, animations, films, guidelines, handouts, presentations, and more.

Web site: https://uktraumacouncil.org/resources?cn-reloaded=1

INDIA

This essential resource provides a fundamental introduction for individuals grappling with the complexities of posttraumatic stress disorder (PTSD) in different states in India. While not exhaustive, it offers a diverse array of support options for those seeking assistance.

Web Sites

Below is a diverse and thorough compilation of Web sites addressing subjects concerning trauma and posttraumatic stress disorder (PTSD).

Royal College of Psychiatrists

Comprehensive page in Hindi about posttraumatic stress disorder, how it manifests as a normal response to trauma, misconceptions surrounding PTSD, treatment and coping tips.

Web site: https://www.rcpsych.ac.uk/mental-health/translations/hindi/post-traumatic-stress-disorder-(ptsd)

Banega Swasth India: जानें क्या है पोस्ट-ट्रॉमैटिक स्ट्रेस डिसिऑर्डर (PTSD)?, लक्षण और बचाव

Web site in Hindi describing PTSD, symptoms, diagnosis, and treatment

Web site: https://swachhindia.ndtv.com/mental-health-explained-what-is-post-traumatic-stress-disorder-hindi-62752/

Alpha Healing Centre

Web site explaining what trauma is, lists different types, and shows examples.

Web site: https://alphahealingcenter.in/trauma-ptsd/

Abhasa Rehab and Wellness

Addiction and mental disorders treatment center

Phone: +91 737 364 4444 / +91 86220 66666

Location: 500/3, 4,5, Kannapiran Mills Rd, Sowri Palayam, Coimbatore, Tamil Nadu 641028

Web site: https://abhasa.in/

Their page on PTSD: https://abhasa.in/post-traumatic-stress-disorder-treatment-in-tamilnadu/

Navbharat Times

Blog post in Hindi about PTSD.

Web site: https://navbharattimes.indiatimes.com/lifestyle/health/what-is-post-traumatic-stress-disorder-its-symptoms-and-treatment/articleshow/71009675.cms

Drishti IAS

Web site in Hindi on PTSD and the role of cerebellum.

Web site: https://www.drishtiias.com/hindi/daily-updates/prelims-facts/post-traumatic-stress-disorder-ptsd-and-cerebellum

Recovery

List of addiction and mental health treatment centers in India.

Web site: https://recovery.com/india/

Harvard T.H. Chan School of Public Health—Viswanath Lab

Web page in Hindi providing tips on how to improve mental health.

Web site: https://www.hsph.harvard.edu/viswanathlab/mental-well-being-hindi/

Cadabam's Hospitals

Treatment center for PTSD patients.

Web site: https://www.cadabamshospitals.com/ptsd/

Neurocon Inc

Lists medications used to treat PTSD.

Web site: https://www.neuroconinc.com/medicines-for-post-traumatic-stress-disorder/

Videos

ट्रॉमा (PTSD) से कैसे निकिलें बाहर? | Post Traumatic Stress Disorder in Hindi

> Link: https://youtu.be/ln6a_VeaCLs?si=o1d04YWcChfKTD7R

Post-traumatic Stress Disorder Kya Hota Hai? (in Hindi)

> A short video of 1.5 min covering an overview of PTSD in Hindi

> Link: https://youtu.be/QnU3Lrc7Uio?si=TlFvdrTRG8q1HPZ9

What Is Post Traumatic Stress Disorder PTSD - In Hindi by Dr Rajiv Sharma Psychiatrist

> Link: https://youtu.be/ARe12gKGt_A?si=VacfzYLzoqPs7L_X

Books

The following lists invaluable resources in the form of books that delve into the topics of trauma, posttraumatic stress disorder (PTSD), and the path to healing.

> *Transcending Trauma: Healing Complex PTSD with Internal Family Systems* by Frank Anderson

> *Recovery from Gaslighting & Narcissistic Abuse, Codependency & Complex PTSD (3 in 1): Emotional Abuse, People-Pleasing and Trauma vs. Emotional Regulation, Mindfulness, Independence and Self-Caring* by Don Barlow

> *Getting Unstuck from PTSD: Using Cognitive Processing Therapy to Guide Your Recovery* by Patricia A. Resick, Shannon Wiltsey Stirman, and Stefanie T. LoSavio

> *Healing Anxiety: A Tibetan Medicine Guide to Healing Anxiety, Stress and PTSD* by Mary Friedman Ryan

> *Guide to Understanding Complex-PTSD* by Moreen Jordan

Helplines

National Commission for Women: a country-wide 24/7 helpline for providing emergency response to women affected by violence

> Phone: 7827 1701 70

> Web site: http://www.ncw.nic.in/helplines

Kiran: 24/7 National Toll free Mental Health Rehabilitation Helpline

Phone: 1800 599 0019

Address: National Institute of Mental Health Rehabilitation, Purana Zila Panchayat Bhawan, Luniya Chauraha, Mandi Road Sehore - 466001

Web site: https://nimhr.ac.in/

MPower Mind Matters: 24/7 Free Mental Health Support Helpline

Phone: 1800 120 820050

Locations: Mumbai, Bengaluru, Kolkata, Pune, Delhi, Virar

Web site: https://mpowerminds.com/oneonone

ND Prana Lifeline: provides free, immediate support for everyone with topics including anxiety, depression, relationships and thoughts of suicide. Lifeline active country-wide between 09:30 a.m. to 6:00 p.m. IST

Phone: 1 800 121 203040 or +91 84895 12307

Address: Nitya Gurukula, "Devi Durai," 53-54, Sri Lakshmwhoi Nagar, Sowripalayam, Coimbatore Tamil Nadu

Web site: https://ngchandrancharities.org/

Parivarthan Counselling Helpline: free anonymous telephone helpline that is serviced by multilingual trained counselors who listen and help anyone in emotional distress. Helpline active from Monday to Friday, 1 p.m. to 10 p.m. IST

Phone: +91 767 660 2602

Address: 1st Floor, # 3310, 8th Cross, 13th Main, HAL 2nd Stage, Bangalore 560 008

Web site: https://parivarthan.org/counselling-helpline/

Vandrevala Foundation: free all-India 24/7 emergency mental health helpline

Phone: +91 9999 666 555 (also available on WhatsApp)

Web site: https://www.vandrevalafoundation.com/free-counseling

Jeevan Aastha Helpline: suicide prevention and mental health counseling helpline

Phone: 1800 233 3330

Address: Jeevan Aastha, S.P. Office, Police Headquarters, Sector 27, Gandhinagar- 382027

Web site: https://www.jeevanaastha.com/

Samaritans Mumbai: helpline providing anonymous emotional support for those who are stressed, distressed, depressed, or suicidal. Helpline active 4 p.m. through 10 p.m. IST (all days). Can also correspond via Gmail

Phone: +91 84229 84528 / +91 84229 84529 / +91 84229 84530

Gmail: talk2samaritans@gmail.com

Address: 402, Jasmine, Opposite Kala Kendra, Dadasaheb Phalke Road, Dadar (E) Mumbai 400014

Additional resources:

Professional Help: they also offer a free service with a counselor. Call +91-84229-84527 between 10 a.m. and 4 p.m. IST (Monday to Friday) for an appointment.

Face To Face: Female callers can meet a volunteer at the center and talk face-to-face in complete confidence. Face-to-face befriending is available every Monday, Thursday, and Saturday from 4 p.m. to 7 p.m. IST for female callers. No appointment needed.

Web site: https://www.samaritansmumbai.org/

Voice That Cares: pan-India free public helpline that provides psychosocial counselling support to individuals for mental health and well-being. Open time: English, Hindi and Telugu—9 a.m. to 9 p.m. IST dailyland Gujarati, Tamil, and Kannada—4 p.m. to 9 p.m. IST daily

Phone: 8448-8448-45

Address: 2972, 1st Floor, 17th Cross, Off K.R. Road, Banashankari 2nd Stage, Bangalore, KA (560070)

Web site: https://www.rocf.org/voice-that-cares/

iCALL: offers free telephone and email-based counseling services, to individuals in emotional and psychological distress, across age, language, gender, sexual orientation, and issues. Available Monday to Saturday: 10:00 a.m. to 8:00 p.m. IST.

Phone: 9152987821

Web site: https://icallhelpline.org/

Pukar Foundation: emotional support helpline that provides confidential and nonjudgmental support to anyone in crisis. Active daily 10 a.m. to 2 p.m. IST.

Phone: 966 389 6669

Web site: https://www.pukarfoundation.org/

National Institute of Mental Health and Neurosciences: 24/7 free helpline for psychosocial support and mental health services during disasters.

Phone: 080–4611 0007

Address: Hosur Road, Near Bangalore Milk Dairy, Bengluru, Karnataka 5600029

Web site: https://nimhans.ac.in/pssmhs-helpline/

APPENDIX: POTENTIAL PHARMACOLOGICAL TREATMENTS FOR POSTTRAUMATIC STRESS DISORDER

Pharmacological treatments are available to assist individuals in managing and overcoming posttraumatic stress disorder (PTSD). These medications, such as selective serotonin reuptake inhibitors (SSRIs) and serotonin-norepinephrine reuptake inhibitors (SNRIs), work by altering neurotransmitter levels in the brain to alleviate symptoms of anxiety, depression, and intrusive thoughts associated with PTSD. Additionally, non-FDA-approved medications like prazosin may target specific symptoms such as nightmares. While pharmacotherapy can be an essential component of PTSD treatment, it is often combined with psychotherapy approaches like cognitive-behavioral therapy (CBT), eye movement desensitization and reprocessing (EMDR), and group therapy to address both the biological and psychological aspects of the disorder. Consulting with a healthcare provider or mental health specialist is crucial to developing a comprehensive treatment plan tailored to the individual's needs and preferences.

The following drugs work in various mechanisms to aid individuals experiencing posttraumatic stress disorder (PTSD) or PTSD-like symptoms. The effectiveness of these medications differs greatly, and many are not recommended for the treatment of PTSD in most cases. Generally, antidepressant medications help to raise the brain neurotransmitter called serotonin, alleviating the psychological, cognitive, and somatic symptoms of PTSD. They also target other problems that are often related to trauma, which can include depression and anxiety. Anticonvulsants are traditionally used to address epilepsy, but their properties have been found to also be effective in addressing adverse PTSD symptoms. Benzodiazepines have not shown clinical efficacy in relieving PTSD symptoms, other than in cases where severe dissociative symptoms are present.

SELECTIVE SEROTONIN REUPTAKE INHIBITORS (SSRIS)

Selective serotonin reuptake inhibitors (SSRIs) are a class of psychiatric medications primarily utilized for their antidepressant properties. Their efficacy extends beyond depression to encompass anxiety disorders, obsessive-compulsive disorder, and posttraumatic stress disorder (PTSD). In the treatment of PTSD, SSRIs are considered first-line pharmacological agents due to their favorable side effect profile, ease of use, and demonstrated effectiveness in alleviating core symptoms.

Mechanism of Action

SSRIs function by inhibiting the reuptake of serotonin, a neurotransmitter implicated in mood regulation, anxiety modulation, emotional responses, and stress response. By blocking the serotonin reuptake transporters, SSRIs increase how much extracellular concentration serotonin is available in the synaptic cleft, thereby enhancing neurotransmission. This mechanism is believed to contribute to the alleviation of symptoms associated with PTSD, such as intrusive thoughts, hyperarousal, and mood disturbances.

Combination with Other Treatments

SSRIs can be used as monotherapy in PTSD treatment or combined with psychotherapy modalities such as cognitive-behavioral therapy (CBT) or eye movement desensitization and reprocessing (EMDR) for collaborative effects.

Effectiveness

Clinical studies and meta-analyses have consistently demonstrated the efficacy of SSRIs in reducing the severity of PTSD symptoms and improving overall functioning. Individual responses to SSRIs may vary, necessitating careful monitoring and adjustment of medication regimens based on treatment response and tolerability. Moreover, SSRIs have been shown to enhance response to psychotherapeutic interventions, such as exposure therapy, when used in combination. According to research, over half of the patients that are being treated with selective serotonin reuptake inhibitors (SSRIs) will experience at least a 30% decrease in their PTSD symptoms.

Administration Guidelines

SSRIs are typically administered orally in the form of tablets or capsules. Dosage initiation often begins at a low-to-moderate level, gradually titrating upward based on individual response and tolerability. Patients should adhere to prescribed dosing schedules and avoid abrupt discontinuation to prevent withdrawal symptoms or recurrence of psychiatric symptoms.

Additional Considerations

While generally well-tolerated, SSRIs can cause adverse effects such as gastrointestinal disturbances, headache, insomnia, and sexual dysfunction. Monitoring for adverse effects and conducting regular follow-up assessments are crucial aspects of managing patients receiving SSRIs. Additionally, SSRIs carry a risk of serotonin syndrome, a potentially life-threatening condition characterized by agitation, confusion, fever, and autonomic instability.

Example of SSRI

Fluoxetine

Fluoxetine is an antidepressant that can be further classified into the family of drugs known as selective serotonin reuptake inhibitors (SSRIs). Among antidepressants, SSRIs are considered first-class medications to treat PTSD. This, however, differs on an individual basis due to family history and individual history of side effects, comorbidities, and response. Currently, only SSRIs sertraline and paroxetine are approved by the Food and Drug Administration (FDA) for the treatment of PTSD. Furthermore, patients with posttraumatic stress disorder (PTSD) commonly present psychological, cognitive, and somatic symptoms, which can include mood disturbances, fatigue, night sweats, sleep disturbances, and memory or concentration difficulties. The mechanism of action of SSRIs includes blocking the reuptake of serotonin, a biological amine, and neurotransmitter. In other words, it blocks the reuptake transporter protein found in the presynaptic terminal, thereby preventing serotonin uptake into the presynaptic neurons. Overall, it works to increase the activity of serotonin to alleviate psychological symptoms. This drug can also be used to treat other illnesses, such as bulimia nervosa, obsessive-compulsive disorder (OCD), premenstrual dysphoric disorder (PMDD), depression, and panic disorder. It is not an over-the-counter drug, meaning it is only available with a doctor's prescription. The product can be found in various dosage forms, including capsule (normal and delayed release), syrup, tablet, and solution.

It is, however, important to note that fluoxetine has a long half-life, where it is two to three days and four to sixteen days for the parent drug and its metabolite form, respectively. Thus, the drug dosage is delicate and must be adjusted with caution in patients with impaired renal or hepatic function to prevent extending the drug's half-life for patients who require long-term therapy. Moreover, common adverse effects of fluoxetine include nausea, insomnia, and tremors. The pharmacokinetics of fluoxetine is well-characterized. The peak plasma concentration is achieved within six to eight hours of oral administration of the drug. It is metabolized by isoenzyme part of the cytochrome P450 system in the liver, such as CYP2D6. As such, drug-drug interactions must be carefully evaluated, especially if fluoxetine is used in conjunction with other liver-metabolized drugs, including CYP2C9, 2D6, and 3A3/4 enzyme inhibitors. Moreover, if SSRIs are ineffective or not well-tolerated, then serotonin and norepinephrine reuptake inhibitors (SNRIs) can be considered as a second line of treatment.

PRAZOSIN

Prazosin is a drug that was initially recognized for its role in hypertension management. Prazosin is FDA-approved for the treatment of hypertension alone or in combination with other antihypertensive agents. Other diseases, however, such as benign prostatic hypertrophy), pheochromocytoma, and scorpion envenomation also can be addressed by the use of Prazosin. Notably, Prazosin has garnered attention for its efficacy in alleviating symptoms associated with posttraumatic stress disorder (PTSD). The drug has the mechanism of action of an alpha-1 antagonist. The antagonism of alpha-1 receptors leads to a reduction in adrenergic activity within the CNS. As such, Prazosin may help to alleviate nightmares and sleep disturbances commonly experienced by individuals with PTSD.

Prozasin has many risks including its associations with orthostatic hypotension and a pronounced first-dose phenomenon, however, prazosin's efficacy in mitigating sleep disturbances and nightmares in PTSD patients has been substantiated. Clinical protocols often initiate oral doses of Prozasin nightly, with subsequent titration based on individual response. Notably, gender-based variations in dosage requirements have been observed, with women typically necessitating lower doses than men. While predominantly administered at bedtime, some therapeutic regimens may include daytime doses to optimize its effects. In the realm of PTSD, prazosin is a promising treatment in its ability to modulate the adrenergic system and ameliorate sleep disturbances.

Mechanism of Action

Prazosin belongs to a class of medications known as alpha-1 adrenergic blockers. Its primary mechanism of action involves blocking the alpha-1 receptors found on blood vessels and certain smooth muscle cells, leading to vasodilation and decreased peripheral vascular resistance. In the context of PTSD, Prazosin's ability to block alpha-1 receptors in the brainstem may also help reduce the hyperarousal and nightmares associated with the disorder, although the exact mechanism remains under investigation.

Effectiveness in PTSD Treatment

Numerous studies and clinical trials have demonstrated the efficacy of Prazosin in reducing the frequency and intensity of nightmares and improving overall sleep quality in individuals with PTSD. While the precise mechanisms underlying Prazosin's effects on PTSD symptoms are not fully understood, its ability to modulate noradrenergic activity in the CNS is thought to play a role. It is important to note that responses to Prazosin may vary among individuals, and not all patients with PTSD experience significant symptom improvement with this medication.

Combination with Other Treatments

Prazosin is often used as an adjunctive therapy in combination with other pharmacological agents or psychotherapeutic interventions for PTSD. When used alongside SSRIs or other antidepressants, Prazosin may complement the effects of these medications, particularly in addressing sleep-related symptoms. Additionally, combining Prazosin with evidence-based psychotherapies such as cognitive-behavioral therapy (CBT) or exposure therapy may enhance overall treatment outcomes by targeting both the physiological and psychological aspects of PTSD.

Administration Guidelines

Prazosin is typically administered orally in tablet form, with dosages tailored to each individual's needs and tolerability. Treatment initiation typically involves starting at a low dose, with gradual titration upward as necessary to achieve optimal therapeutic effects. It is recommended to take Prazosin at bedtime to minimize the risk of orthostatic hypotension, a potential side effect characterized by a sudden drop in blood pressure upon standing. Regular monitoring of blood pressure and symptoms is essential during Prazosin therapy to ensure efficacy and safety.

Additional Considerations

While generally well-tolerated, Prazosin may cause side effects such as dizziness, light-headedness, fatigue, and nasal congestion, particularly when initiating treatment or adjusting dosages. Orthostatic hypotension, characterized by a sudden decrease in blood pressure upon standing, is another potential concern, especially in elderly patients or those taking other medications that affect blood pressure. Patients should be advised to rise slowly from a sitting or lying position to minimize this risk. Additionally, Prazosin may interact with certain medications, including other antihypertensive agents, necessitating close monitoring and potential dose adjustments.

ANTIDEPRESSANT MEDICATIONS

Antidepressant medications are a class of pharmacological agents widely used in the treatment of various mental health conditions, including depression, anxiety disorders, and posttraumatic stress disorder (PTSD).

Mechanism of Action

Antidepressants exert their therapeutic effects through various mechanisms, depending on the specific class of medication. Selective serotonin reuptake inhibitors (SSRIs), serotonin-norepinephrine reuptake inhibitors (SNRIs), tricyclic antidepressants (TCAs), and monoamine oxidase inhibitors (MAOIs) are among the most commonly prescribed antidepressants. While the precise mechanisms of action differ, these medications generally work by modulating neurotransmitter levels in the brain, particularly serotonin, norepinephrine, and dopamine. In the context of PTSD, antidepressants may help alleviate symptoms such as depressed mood, anxiety, and intrusive thoughts by restoring neurotransmitter balance and enhancing neuroplasticity.

Effectiveness in PTSD Treatment

Antidepressants, particularly SSRIs and SNRIs, have been extensively studied for their efficacy in treating PTSD symptoms. Clinical trials and meta-analyses have consistently demonstrated the effectiveness of these medications in reducing the severity of PTSD symptoms, improving overall functioning, and enhancing quality of life. While individual responses to antidepressants may vary, they are considered first-line pharmacological agents in the treatment of PTSD, especially when symptoms are severe or persistent.

Combination with Other Treatments

Antidepressants are often used as monotherapy in PTSD treatment, but they can also be combined with psychotherapeutic interventions for synergistic effects. Cognitive-behavioral therapy (CBT), prolonged exposure (PE) therapy, and eye movement desensitization and reprocessing (EMDR) are examples of evidence-based psychotherapies that may complement the effects of antidepressant medications. Combination therapy approaches address both the neurobiological and psychological aspects of PTSD, potentially leading to better treatment outcomes.

Administration Guidelines

Antidepressants are typically administered orally, commonly available in tablet or capsule formulations. Dosage initiation and titration vary depending on the specific medication, individual patient factors, and treatment response. It is essential for patients to adhere to prescribed dosing schedules and to continue treatment for an adequate duration to experience maximum benefit. Regular monitoring by healthcare providers is necessary to assess treatment response, manage side effects, and adjust medication regimens as needed.

Additional Considerations

While generally well-tolerated, antidepressants may cause side effects such as gastrointestinal disturbances, headache, insomnia, and sexual dysfunction. Patients should be educated about potential side effects, and healthcare providers should monitor for their occurrence during treatment. Additionally, antidepressants carry a risk of discontinuation syndrome, especially when abruptly stopping medication. Patients should be gradually tapered off antidepressants under medical supervision to minimize withdrawal symptoms.

Examples of Antidepressant Medications

This is not an exhaustive list of antidepressant medications. Please consult with medical professionals to learn more about available antidepressant medication treatment plans.

Sertraline

Sertraline is an antidepressant, which can be further classified into the family of drugs known as selective serotonin reuptake inhibitors (SSRIs). Among antidepressants, SSRIs are considered first-class medications to treat PTSD. This, however, differs on an individual basis due to family history and individual history of side effects, comorbidities, and response. Currently, only SSRIs sertraline and paroxetine are approved by the Food and Drug Administration (FDA) for the treatment of PTSD. Furthermore, patients with posttraumatic stress disorder (PTSD) commonly present psychological, cognitive, and somatic symptoms, which can include mood disturbances, fatigue, night sweats, sleep disturbances, and memory or concentration difficulties. The mechanism of action of SSRIs includes blocking the reuptake of serotonin, a biological amine, and neurotransmitter. In other words, it blocks the reuptake transporter protein found in the presynaptic terminal, thereby preventing serotonin uptake into the presynaptic neurons. Overall, it works to increase the activity of serotonin to alleviate psychological symptoms. This drug can also be used to treat other illnesses, such as bulimia nervosa, obsessive-compulsive disorder (OCD), premenstrual dysphoric disorder (PMDD), depression, and panic disorder. It is not an over-counter drug, meaning it is only available with a doctor's prescription. The product can be found in various dosage forms, including capsule (normal and delayed release), syrup, tablet, and solution.

Sertraline is effective in 50% of patients with PTSD or PTSD-like symptoms. Moreover, patients exhibited improvement in symptoms regarding depression and OCD relative to the control group. It is successful in alleviating symptoms of depression, and in reducing perfectionist attitudes, ineffectiveness, a lack of interoceptive awareness, as well as anxiety.

Overall, sertraline is a well-tolerated drug with minimal patients who reported experiencing side effects at the beginning of their treatments. A caveat associated with sertraline is that it may be more effective in an outpatient setting compared to an inpatient setting. Additionally, the use of sertraline with grapefruit juice may increase the risk of experiencing certain side effects, which should be treated with caution. Drug-drug interactions are common with sertraline, and as such, the treatment should be closely monitored and consulted with a physician, pharmacist, or other healthcare professionals. Moreover, it should be noted that interventions such as cognitive-processing therapy, cognitive-behavioral therapy (CBT), eye movement desensitization, and reprocessing or narrative exposure therapy are more effective than the use of sertraline alone for patients with PTSD. As such, it is encouraged for patients to consult their healthcare professionals about the most effective treatment for PTSD.

Tricyclic Antidepressants

Tricyclic antidepressants (TCAs) are a class of drugs commonly used to treat major depressive disorders (MDDs). Their mechanism of action is well-studied, where they inhibit neurotransmitter reuptake, such as serotonin and norepinephrine. They help regulate mood, attention, and pain in patients. As such, they are useful in treating migraine prophylaxis, obsessive-compulsive disorder (OCD), diabetic neuropathy, and postherpetic neuralgia. Imipramine is the first TCA created, initially for the function as an antipsychotic, but its antidepressant effects were observed, which caused the subsequent development of other TCAs (e.g., Amitriptyline, desipramine, doxepin, etc.). TCAs are named "tricyclic" as their chemical structure contains three rings. It is available in various dosage forms, including oral tablets, capsules, and solutions. It is less common to administer TCAs through intravenous (IV) injections, although it is possible. There are also topical creams or transdermal patches that contain TCAs, but oral administration remains the standard and allows for the most potent effects.

TCAs exhibit similar efficacy with selective serotonin reuptake inhibitors (SSRIs), however, they are considered a second-line treatment for MDD as they have a higher risk of causing side effects, have anticholinergic activity, and have a lower tolerance for overdose. The pharmacokinetics of TCAs are well-characterized, which is crucial in the development of dosing strategies and for predicting drug-drug interactions. PCAs reach peak plasma concentrations within two to eight hours after oral administration, and their bioavailability varies from 40%–50%. The consumption of food can affect the absorption rate, especially foods that contain higher lipophilicity (ex. amitriptyline). Most TCAs are metabolized by cytochrome P450 (CYP) enzymes, such as CYP2D6 and CYP2C19. Importantly, a caveat of TCAs is that they can affect the availability of other chemicals such as histamine and acetylcholine, subsequently affecting other nerve signaling events. This leads to various potential side effects, including drowsiness, difficulty urinating, blurred vision, sweating, palpitations, and a change in appetite. As such, the use of TCAs should proceed with caution.

NOVEL ANTIPSYCHOTICS

Novel antipsychotics, also known as second-generation antipsychotics (SGAs) or atypical antipsychotics, have gained recognition for their broad spectrum of pharmacological effects beyond the treatment of psychotic disorders. In recent years, their use in the management of posttraumatic stress disorder (PTSD) has garnered attention, particularly for their potential to target specific symptoms such as agitation, mood instability, and intrusive thoughts. This appendix explores the mechanisms, effectiveness, administration guidelines, and additional considerations associated with the use of novel antipsychotics in the context of treating PTSD.

Mechanism of Action

Novel antipsychotics exert their therapeutic effects through complex interactions with various neurotransmitter systems in the brain, including dopamine, serotonin, and glutamate. Unlike first-generation antipsychotics, which primarily block dopamine receptors, novel antipsychotics have a broader receptor profile, with varying affinities for serotonin receptors. This serotonin-dopamine antagonism is believed to contribute to their efficacy in alleviating symptoms of psychosis, mood disorders, and PTSD by modulating neurotransmitter activity and restoring neurochemical balance in key brain regions implicated in PTSD pathophysiology.

Effectiveness in PTSD Treatment

Clinical studies and case reports have suggested the potential efficacy of novel antipsychotics, such as quetiapine, risperidone, and olanzapine, in reducing the severity of PTSD symptoms, particularly in cases where standard treatments have been ineffective or poorly tolerated. These medications may help alleviate symptoms of hyperarousal, irritability, and mood instability, thereby improving overall functioning and quality of life. It's important to note that the evidence for the use of novel antipsychotics in PTSD remains limited compared to other pharmacological agents, and further research is needed to elucidate their role in treatment.

Combination with Other Treatments

Novel antipsychotics are often used as adjunctive therapy in combination with other pharmacological agents or psychotherapeutic interventions for PTSD. When used alongside antidepressants or mood stabilizers, they may augment the effects of these medications, particularly in managing symptoms such as agitation, aggression, and impulsivity. Additionally, novel antipsychotics can complement evidence-based psychotherapies such as cognitive-behavioral therapy (CBT) or exposure therapy by addressing specific symptom clusters that may not fully respond to psychotherapy alone.

Administration Guidelines

Novel antipsychotics are typically administered orally, available in tablet, capsule, or liquid formulations. Dosage initiation and titration vary depending on the specific medication, individual patient factors, and treatment response. It is essential for patients to adhere to prescribed dosing schedules and to continue treatment for an adequate duration to assess efficacy. Regular monitoring by healthcare providers is necessary to assess treatment response, manage side effects, and adjust medication regimens as needed.

Additional Considerations

While generally well tolerated, novel antipsychotics may cause side effects such as sedation, weight gain, metabolic disturbances, and extrapyramidal symptoms (e.g., tremor, stiffness, and involuntary movements). Patients should be educated about potential side effects, and healthcare providers should monitor for their occurrence during treatment. Additionally, novel antipsychotics carry a risk of rare but serious adverse effects, including neuroleptic malignant syndrome (NMS) and tardive dyskinesia (TD), necessitating vigilant monitoring and timely intervention if suspected.

MONOAMINE OXIDASE INHIBITORS (MAOI)

Brofaromine is a selective monoamine oxidase inhibitor (MAOI) that also has serotonin reuptake inhibitory properties. Its properties hold promise in treating patients with a variety of psychiatric disorders while producing less severe anticholinergic side effects. Monoamine oxidase inhibitors (MAOIs) are a class of drugs that inhibit the enzyme monoamine oxidase which is expressed in neurons. They increase the concentration of amines in the cytoplasms of neuronal cells as well as in the synaptic clefts between them. It is suggested that MAOIs are effective in treating depression and anxiety disorders by elevating levels of catecholamines and serotonin. Individuals taking MAOIs however must follow a tyramine diet to avoid the side effects of potentially lethal levels of hypertension. While MAOIs are FDA-approved for the treatment of major depressive disorder, they are one of the least commonly prescribed antidepressants due to safety concerns around food and drug interactions.

Trials with brofaromine as well as other monoamine oxidase inhibitors such as phenelzine and moclobemide demonstrate efficacy for the treatment of posttraumatic stress disorder (PTSD). They demonstrated a decrease of intrusive, but not avoidance, or depressive symptoms of PTSD. This is because the depressive symptoms associated with PTSD may be more treatment-resistant than traditional depressive syndromes. In other trials, however, Brofaromine did not show superiority in comparison to a placebo for reducing PTSD symptoms. Specifically, half of the brofaromine-treated patients continued to meet the criteria for PTSD at the end of the trial. Currently, brofaromine is not available for market and research use. Side effects of brofaromine include dry mouth, dizziness, tremor, hypomania, anxiety, and memory problems.

LITHIUM

Lithium is an element that influences the CNS by modulating various neurotransmitters. The primary target symptoms of lithium are mania and unstable mood. These neurotransmitters include serotonin, dopamine, norepinephrine, acetylcholine, and gamma-aminobutyric acid (GABA). It was the first mood stabilizer and is still the first-line treatment option but is underutilized due to being outdated. Lithium is effective for addressing manic episodes in bipolar disorder. Lithium is also often effectively used to augment antidepressant treatments as well as to manage impulse control and aggression issues.

The use of lithium to manage posttraumatic stress disorder (PTSD) is limited. The existing literature on lithium's effectiveness in PTSD is sparse. One study that involves combat veterans resistant to conventional treatments demonstrates lithium's effectiveness in improving anxiety, anger, irritability, and insomnia.

A problem with the use of lithium, however, is its narrow therapeutic range. Toxicity easily occurs when lithium levels are unregulated and can cause damage to the kidneys, thyroid, and heart. The difficulty of therapeutic drug monitoring combined with the challenges of compliance associated with PTSD makes lithium an undesirable treatment option for symptom relief in PTSD.

ANTICONVULSANTS

Carbamazepine and valproic acid are some of the most common anti-convulsants, a class of drugs originally designed to manage and prevent seizures and epilepsy. These drugs, however, have become important in addressing various other neurological and psychiatric conditions. Anticonvulsants act by modulating the excitability of neurons, often through interactions with ion channels and neurotransmitter pathways. Carbamazepine and valproic acid have been historically used to manage epilepsy. More recently, however, these drugs have been implicated in the treatment of posttraumatic stress disorder (PTSD), demonstrating potential benefits in alleviating intrusive symptoms and emotional lability while reducing hypervigilance and startle response.

Carbamazepine, FDA-approved for epilepsy, trigeminal neuralgia, and bipolar I disorder, involves the modulation of voltage-gated sodium channels (VGSC), limiting action potentials, and reducing synaptic transmission. In PTSD, carbamazepine's anticonvulsants are suggested to contribute to mitigating exaggerated fear responses, mood instability, anger, and aggression when remembering traumatic experiences.

Valproic acid is also FDA-approved for the treatment of epilepsy, bipolar disorder, and migraines. Anticonvulsants like valproic acid have been introduced for mood stabilization, reflecting their antikindling properties. While research on their efficacy in PTSD is limited, evidence suggests improvement in intrusive symptoms and emotional lability. Valproic acid, like carbamazepine, may address limbic structures' sensitization, contributing to exaggerated reactions to stressors in PTSD.

These anticonvulsants, with their established roles in neurological and psychiatric disorders, present a novel approach to PTSD treatment. Further research is needed to demonstrate the potential for carbamazepine and valproic acid to mitigate trauma-associated symptoms.

BENZODIAZEPINES

Alprazolam is a benzodiazepine that has anxiolytic properties and finds application in various aspects of psychiatric care. Drugs in the benzodiazepine family exert their effects by binding to the GABA-A receptor, a neuropeptide receptor with various subunits. The inhibition of the alpha-1 subunits mediates sedation, amnesia, and ataxic effects. Meanwhile, the inhibition of the alpha-2 and alpha-3 subunits contributes to anxiolytic and muscle-relaxing effects.

In the context of posttraumatic stress disorder (PTSD), alprazolam's utility has been explored in controlled trials revealing a reduction in overall anxiety ratings, yet no discernible changes in core PTSD symptoms. Other benzodiazepines such as clonazepam have also failed to suppress auditory startle responses in PTSD patients and do not alter the long-term trajectory of PTSD symptoms. Despite the intuitive inclination to employ benzodiazepines for the chronic anxiety implicated in PTSD, limited evidence supports these hypotheses. Considerations for initiating benzodiazepine treatment in PTSD necessitate careful evaluation, factoring in the risk of abuse and the potential for withdrawal to exacerbate PTSD symptoms. In some cases, however, benzodiazepines are useful in treating the severe dissociative symptoms present in refractory PTSD.

INDEX